Do They Grow Out of It?

Long-Term Outcomes of Childhood Disorders

Do They Grow Out of It?

Long-Term Outcomes of Childhood Disorders

Edited by
Lily Hechtman, M.D., F.R.C.P.C.

Washington, DC
London, England

Copyright © 1996 American Psychiatric Press, Inc.
ALL RIGHTS RESERVED
Manufactured in the United States of America on acid-free paper
99 98 97 96   4 3 2 1
American Psychiatric Press, Inc.
1400 K Street, N.W., Washington, DC   20005

Library of Congress Cataloging-in-Publication Data
Do they grow out of it? : long-term outcomes of childhood disorders /
  edited by Lily Hechtman.
      p.   cm.
  Includes bibliographical references and index.
  ISBN 0-88048-703-8
  1. Child psychopathology—Longitudinal studies.   2. Adjustment
(Psychology)—Longitudinal studies.   3. Mental illness—Prognosis.
I. Hechtman, Lily Trokenberg.
  [DNLM: 1. Child Behavior Disorders.   2. Mental Disorders—in
infancy & childhood.   3. Longitudinal Studies.   WS 350.6 D631 1996]
RJ499.D59   1996
618.92'89—dc20
DNLM/DLC
for Library of Congress   95-46924
                                                              CIP

British Library Cataloguing in Publication Data
A CIP record is available from the British Library.

Contents

Contributors

Joseph H. Beitchman, M.D., F.R.C.P.C., D.A.B.P.N.
Head, Child and Family Studies Centre, Clarke Institute of
Psychiatry; and Professor, Departments of Psychiatry and
Preventative Medicine and Biostatistics, University of Toronto,
Toronto, Ontario, Canada

Kathryn J. Bennett, M.Sc.
Member, Centre for the Studies of Children at Risk, Chedoke
Division, Chedoke-McMaster Hospitals and Faculty of Health
Sciences, McMaster University, and Assistant Professor,
Department of Clinical Epidemiology and Biostatistics,
McMaster University, Hamilton, Ontario, Canada

Joseph Biederman, M.D.
Chief, Pediatric Psychopharmacology Unit, Massachusetts
General Hospital; and Professor of Psychiatry, Harvard Medical
School, Boston, Massachusetts

E.B. Brownlie, B.Sc.
Research Associate, Child and Family Studies Centre, Clarke
Institute of Psychiatry, Toronto, Canada

Valerie Del Medico, M.D.
Private practice, Columbus, Ohio

Stephen V. Faraone, Ph.D.
Director of Research, Pediatric Psychopharmacology Unit,
Massachusetts General Hospital; and Associate Professor of
Psychology, Department of Psychiatry, Harvard Medical School,
Boston, Massachusetts

Lily Hechtman, M.D., F.R.C.P.C.
Director of Research, Division of Child Psychiatry, and Professor of Pediatrics and Psychiatry, McGill University; and Director of Adolescent Services and Staff Psychiatrist, Montreal Children's Hospital, Montreal, Canada

Kathleen Kiely, B.A.
Research Associate, Pediatric Psychopharmacology Unit, Massachusetts General Hospital, Boston, Massachusetts

Marge C. Lenane, M.S.W.
Senior Research Social Worker, Child Psychiatry Branch, National Institute of Mental Health, Bethesda, Maryland

Henrietta L. Leonard, M.D.
Professor of Psychiatry and Human Behavior, Brown University School of Medicine, Rhode Island Hospital, Providence, Rhode Island

Diane Majcher, M.D., M.S.
Research Associate, Anxiety Disorders Program, Massachusetts General Hospital; and Instructor, Department of Psychiatry, Harvard Medical School, Boston, Massachusetts

David R. Offord, M.D.
Director, Centre for Studies of Children at Risk, Chedoke Division, Chedoke-McMaster Hospitals, and Faculty of Health Sciences, McMaster University; and Professor, Department of Psychiatry, McMaster University, Hamilton, Ontario, Canada

Cynthia R. Pfeffer, M.D.
Professor of Psychiatry, Cornell University Medical College; and Chief, Child Psychiatry Inpatient Unit, New York Hospital—Westchester Division, White Plains, New York

Joanna Pleeter
Child Psychiatry Branch, National Institute of Mental Health, Bethesda, Maryland

Mark H. Pollack, M.D.
Director, Anxiety Disorders Program, Massachusetts General Hospital; and Associate Professor of Psychiatry, Harvard Medical School, Boston, Massachusetts

Gabrielle Weiss, M.D., F.R.C.P.C.
Professor of Psychiatry, University of British Columbia, West Vancouver, British Columbia, Canada

Elizabeth Weller, M.D.
Professor of Psychiatry, Pediatrics, and Neurosciences, Department of Psychiatry, Neuropsychiatric Facility, The Ohio State University, Columbus, Ohio

Ronald Weller, M.D.
Professor of Psychiatry, College of Medicine, The Ohio State University, Columbus, Ohio

John Scott Werry, M.D.
Emeritus Professor of Psychiatry, University of Auckland, Auckland, New Zealand

Preface

Long-term outcome of childhood disorders is becoming increasingly more important as we begin to take a broader, more comprehensive view of childhood disorders: their natural history and developmental impact, their possible multigenerational consequences, and the ability of individuals with childhood disorders to function in later adolescence and adulthood.

In addition, as we have begun to look at long-term outcome of childhood disorders, we have become aware of a multitude of factors that may affect this outcome. Factors pertaining to the child—the age at onset of the condition, its severity, other comorbid conditions, the child's sex and IQ, and his or her physical or neurological health—all seem important in influencing outcome. In addition, factors pertaining to the family, such as socioeconomic status (SES), family composition, mental health of parents, family functioning, and child-rearing practices, also seem to affect outcome. Finally, the impact of treatment on outcome is also crucial because it provides a picture of the long-term efficacy of various treatment approaches.

In the chapters that follow, we have tried to touch upon the major childhood disorders. Each chapter critically reviews available information on long-term outcome of the particular childhood disorder; what factors, particularly treatments, influence this outcome; and what future research or clinical directions appear promising.

Gabrielle Weiss, in the first chapter, "Research Issues in Longitudinal Studies," reviews the importance and value of longitudinal research. She also outlines various types of longitudinal studies with their specific strengths and limitations. The chapter ends with an illustration of how some of these issues were addressed in the prospective 15-year follow-up of hyperactive children.

Lily Hechtman, in Chapter 2, "Attention-Deficit/Hyperactivity Disorder," reviews studies that focus on adolescent and adult outcome in attention-deficit/hyperactivity disorder (ADHD). The studies reveal that adolescent outcome is quite problematic, and the adult outcome can be divided into three distinct groups: a fairly healthy-outcome group; a group with continuing symptoms of the syndrome, resulting in social, emotional, work, and interpersonal problems (most adult ADHD subjects fall into this group); and, finally, a small proportion of adults with childhood ADHD who are seriously psychiatrically or antisocially impaired. Factors that may affect these various outcomes are discussed.

Joseph Biederman, Stephen Faraone, and Kathleen Kiely, in Chapter 3, "Comorbidity in Outcome of Attention-Deficit/Hyperactivity Disorder," outline the possible sources of "artifactual" comorbidity. They then proceed to discuss the evidence of comorbidity in children with ADHD and their relatives. Comorbid conditions, such as major depression, conduct disorder, anxiety disorder, and learning disabilities, are all explored. The authors then outline the evidence of various comorbid conditions in adult ADHD subjects. The chapter ends with a discussion of the implications of comorbidity in the clinical picture, and a discussion of diagnosis, treatment, and prognosis.

David Offord and Kathryn Bennett, in Chapter 4, "Conduct Disorder," explore the evidence of continuity of aggression and violence. They then discuss the outcome of conduct disorder as seen from retrospective and prospective studies, both in clinical or high-risk populations and in the community. Factors that may influence outcome—such as comorbidity, age at onset, and characteristics of the symptomatology, as well as some physiological measures—are also explored. The chapter ends with a detailed description of the effects on long-term outcome of various interventions, such as family therapy, social cognitive treatment, peer- and school-based interventions, and community-centered treatment. Future directions regarding research, prevention, and treatment are also discussed.

Valerie Del Medico, Elizabeth Weller, and Ronald Weller, in Chapter 5, "Childhood Depression," review the distinction between the depressive episode and recurrence of depression. The development and co-occurrence of comorbid conditions are addressed. Factors that impart resilience or vulnerability are reviewed. Specifically, the role of family dysfunction, low self-esteem, and stressful life events are all explored. The effect of treatment of depressed children on adolescent outcome is also discussed.

Cynthia Pfeffer, in Chapter 6, "Suicidal Behavior," reviews previous studies of outcome for children with suicidal behavior and then focuses on the relationship between intervention and outcome. Other factors that influence outcome are also explored. Specifically, factors such as low SES, previous psychiatric inpatient treatment, substance abuse, and previous suicide attempt all tend to increase the risk of future suicidal behavior. The author also discusses the vulnerability of a community sample to suicidal behavior. Finally, the efficacy of prevention programs is addressed. Future research and treatment directions are also explored.

Diane Majcher and Mark Pollack, in Chapter 7, "Childhood Anxiety Disorders," outline the difficulties of studying anxiety disorders in childhood. They then explore the link between childhood and adult anxiety disorders by discussing retrospective studies of the history of childhood anxiety, "top-down" and "bottom-up" studies of families, and studies on the long-term outcome of anxiety and anxiety disorders. Specific conditions, such as behavioral inhibition, separation anxiety disorder, school refusal, panic disorder, overanxious disorder, avoidant disorder, social phobia, phobic disorder, and posttraumatic stress disorder, are also discussed. Studies addressing the efficacy of treatment approaches for these various disorders are described.

Joanna Pleeter, Marge Lenane, and Henrietta Leonard, in Chapter 8, "Obsessive-Compulsive Disorder," provide a brief history of our awareness of this disorder, its phenomenology, and its epidemiology. They then go on to discuss the neurobiology and treatment of obsessive-compulsive disorder (OCD). Early and more recent follow-up studies of adult OCD are reviewed. Similarly, early and more recent pediatric OCD follow-up studies are described. The efficacy of more recent pharmacotherapeutic and behavior treatments are presented, and factors that may influence treatment response are outlined.

John Scott Werry, in Chapter 9, "Pervasive Developmental, Psychotic, and Allied Disorders," outlines DSM-IV definitions and characteristics of autism, Asperger's disorder, and pervasive developmental disorder. The problems of outcome studies of these disorders are described and the various types of outcome are summarized. The effect of treatment on outcome is addressed as well as other factors that may influence outcome, such as severity of the disorder, IQ, language development, and the presence of other physical disorders. The author then addresses schizophrenia in children and adolescents. Again, methodological problems in outcome studies in early-onset schizophrenia are outlined, long-term outcome studies are summarized, and the effect of treatment and other factors on outcome are addressed. Finally, the author explores the issues of bipolar mood disorder in children and adolescents. Factors such as intelligence, premorbid functioning, gender, positive family history, and mixed and cycling forms of the disorder all appear to have affected outcome.

Joseph Beitchman and E. B. Brownlie, in Chapter 10, "Childhood Speech and Language Disorders," describe the various forms of language disorders and their developmental course. The epidemiology of these disorders and their comorbidity with hyperactivity, elective mutism, learning disabilities, autism, and other emotional disorders, such as anxiety and depression, are addressed. Studies involving long-term outcome are described, and factors that may influence this outcome are delineated. Directions for future diagnosis, treatment, and outcome studies are outlined.

Gabrielle Weiss, in Chapter 11, "Clinical Issues in Longitudinal Research," shares her own personal experiences in conducting a 15-year prospective study of children diagnosed with ADHD. The many lessons learned in sharing the lives of these children as they became adolescents and adults are movingly described. Weiss graphically illustrates how people cope, the creative ways they overcome handicaps and adversity, and the dramatic influence sustained by unexpected life events. Three detailed case vignettes of people followed from childhood to adulthood are presented to illustrate her points. These histories leave an indelible picture of people struggling courageously and creatively to adapt and succeed despite adversities. They teach all of us the true meaning of long-term outcome of childhood disorders.

Chapter 1

Research Issues in Longitudinal Studies

Gabrielle Weiss, M.D., F.R.C.P.C.

This chapter outlines and describes the key role of longitudinal studies in promoting our understanding of the course of various conditions and the factors that influence this course. The strengths and weaknesses of various types of longitudinal studies are discussed along with the particular methodological issues that are involved.

▼ Roles of Longitudinal Studies

Determining Adult Outcome

It is only through one of the types of longitudinal studies (to be described) that we can learn the outcome of a childhood disorder. Clinical judgment of outcome without the use of systematic research methodology that employs a control group or a comparison group is

notoriously misleading. It is an interesting piece of historical information that a disorder such as attention-deficit/hyperactivity disorder (ADHD) was thought by clinicians up until the 1970s to be
a childhood disorder that was outgrown sometime during adolescence (Laufer and Denhoff 1957). Later, Laufer (1971) followed
his childhood patients into adulthood by sending letters with questionnaires to 66 parents. Although many parents did not respond,
those who did indicated that their now grown children had frequently become troubled adults. Why pediatricians and child psychiatrists believed at that time that ADHD was "outgrown" is a
mystery. Possibly this belief was related to the fact that one cardinal
symptom—hyperactivity—abated in intensity during adolescence,
or it might have resulted from patients in late adolescence leaving
their pediatricians and child psychiatrists to see family physicians,
so that the former doctors, who had stopped seeing their patients,
were unaware that problems changed but continued. We now know
that most childhood syndromes are not outgrown in childhood,
making more longitudinal studies essential.

Establishing a Relationship Between Child and Adult Psychiatry

Longitudinal studies give us the only method of fitting together the
missing pieces between child and adult disorders. Psychiatry and
child psychiatry are two disciplines with quite different origins.
Child psychiatry, which arose in the United States after World
War I, did not come into being as a result of the curiosity or the
need for knowledge on the part of psychiatrists. Rather, it was the
result of a particular judge in Chicago who felt he had to know why
the juvenile offenders he sentenced had committed their different
offenses. He recognized that several of them seemed to be intellectually delayed, whereas others came from severely troubled families. Through his influence, a practicing obstetrician, Dr. William
Healey, was recruited and began to conduct studies on impaired
children. He carried out these studies under Freud's supervision
and in Binet's clinic in Europe. Healey returned to found the first
Child Guidance Clinic in Chicago, which was soon followed by

many more in other states. These clinics became precursors of our current child psychiatric clinics. This excursion into how child psychiatry came into being probably has a bearing on the fact that child and adult psychiatry have often been, and still are, so unconnected. This has been detrimental to both disciplines. Longitudinal studies and the whole field of developmental psychopathology seeks to redress this.

Determining Changes in Symptomatology and Life Events

The continuities and discontinuities in the nature and intensity of a given syndrome's symptomatology—the change in one individual from year to year as maturation occurs—can only be learned from prospective longitudinal studies. Such changes can teach us what may act to increase risk or to decrease it. For example, the Kauai longitudinal study of perinatal complications showed that poor outcome was related to adverse socioeconomic factors and family disturbance, and that vulnerability to disorder differed for different sexes at different ages (Werner 1989). Similarly, the outcome for institutionalized infants could be ameliorated if the adult women who had been institutionalized in their infancy married a stable partner in adulthood (Rutter 1985). In contrast, Gittelman-Klein et al.'s (1985) prospective longitudinal study found that the continuation of ADHD symptoms into late adolescence was a serious risk factor for drug abuse and antisocial personality disorder.

Determining the Effect on Syndromes of Acute Stressful Life Events

Crises in the lives of troubled children are more common than in the lives of healthy children. When they occur they may affect the course of the disorder and its treatment. For example, Willy was an 8-year-old boy treated for ADHD and doing well on a given dose of methylphenidate. One night his father (an adult with ADHD) lost his temper with his son and locked him out of the house. Willy ran away, was picked up by a child molester, and had unfortunate experiences over several days until found by the police. After this episode Willy's course of ADHD worsened, and his normal dose of methylphenidate no longer improved his core symptoms. He also developed an adjustment disorder with anxiety and depression. Crisis intervention was offered, but it took several years before the child was closer to his previous level of functioning. Jamie was a 9-year-old boy who lived with his single, divorced mother and was diagnosed as having dysthymia. Both had been abandoned by the father several years previously. When the mother remarried a stable person who cared about Jamie, Jamie initially developed a major depression with suicidal ideation and had plans to kill himself by running in front of a bus. This brought Jamie into treatment, and with the help of a caring father figure and therapy, he was able to recover.

Validating the Syndrome

Shaffer and Greenhill (1979) wrote that a childhood syndrome requires validation with respect to predictive validity, consensual validity, and postdictive validity. Predictive validity is present when most subjects have a common outcome. Consensual validity presupposes that a given syndrome has symptoms common to all children who have the syndrome, other than those that define the syndrome. Postdictive validity requires a common cause, or at least common antecedent variables. This clear-cut picture is not generally available for childhood or adult psychopathological syndromes. For example, with respect to ADHD, Biederman et al. (1991) have shown that, for many children with the syndrome, a genetic predisposition exists that interacts with psychosocial factors. This has increased the postdictive validity of the syndrome. Cognitive difficulties such as learning disabilities and lower IQ (the consensual validity for the syndrome) are present over time, as longitudinal studies have shown. The predictive validity from prospective follow-up studies shows similarities for the course of the disorder and the adult outcome.

Thus, longitudinal studies have provided us with evidence for the existence of ADHD as a specific syndrome, from the point of view of predictive consensual and postdictive validity. Verhulst and Koot (1991) pointed out that longitudinal studies are not possible without standardized and reliable assessment procedures, but longitudinal studies not only serve to validate the syndrome, but can also help to evaluate and validate measures used in assessment. In past research we have at times found that popularly used rating scales were flawed in that they measured overlapping syndromes and were not specific for one diagnostic syndrome (e.g., the Connor's Rating Scale for ADHD until it was factor analyzed). Assessment measures are revised over time, and thus require revalidation on healthy samples. Unemployment or poverty in times of recession will change families and therefore the norms of children.

Determining Risk Factors for Outcome

Risk factors that constitute a good versus a poor prognosis give us essential clinical data required by parents, and are essential for determining treatment and prevention. Determination of risk factors may also help us to delineate different overlapping syndromes. In general, comorbidity is a serious risk factor in itself and is receiving much more attention as its prevalence has become increasingly apparent. The failure to look for coexisting conditions has confused longitudinal outcome studies in the past.

Providing Information on Treatment Effects

Longitudinal studies give us essential information for planning treatment in terms of type of treatment and when it is best given. Children with ADHD, or children with major depression or, for that matter, children with most psychopathological disorders are known to be at risk for social rejection and school failure. To avoid these secondary consequences, early effective treatment is important. For children with ADHD, stimulants, educational aid, and family help may be very effective when provided before severe school failure sets in, with consequent lack of motivation for learning.

Aiding in Prevention

Cross-sectional population surveys (Szatmari et al. 1989) can provide us with information about the prevalence of a given syndrome at different ages. ADHD, for example, is present in preschool children but usually only comes to clinical diagnosis in the first 1 to 3 years of elementary school. Screening for ADHD symptoms in kindergarten could serve to flag youngsters at risk for later school failure and behavior problems. Longitudinal surveys can then be used to evaluate the efficacy of various kinds of early intervention for children at risk with respect to their subsequent outcome. Good screening measures can be found to detect any syndrome in preschool or kindergarten before diagnosis. However, little is known about how much effect such early detection has on the seriousness of the subsequent disorder.

Head Start programs became important in the United States in the 1960s. They were designed to prevent school failure for disadvantaged preschool children by providing stimulation before school began. They were at first found to be effective but the positive effect was not lasting, in that the additional stimulation was not continued. Later longitudinal studies discovered that a "sleeper effect" had occurred, which was positive for the children who had been in Head Start programs. Without longitudinal studies these initially hidden benefits, which did not immediately appear, would have been missed. More careful and continuous prospective follow-up on these children over a period of years would have provided even more information regarding when and how the initial benefits wore off and how the later positive benefits took place. In this way the effectiveness of Head Start could have been augmented.

▼ Types of Longitudinal Studies

Anteroceptive Studies

These kinds of studies generally start with a birth cohort that is representative of the population and that is large enough to provide information on the development of specific syndromes, and also on the risk factors for poor outcome. For example, the Kauai study already referred to has been invaluable in demonstrating the interaction of a risk factor such as perinatal difficulties, which was shown to be a risk only when it was associated with socioeconomic and psychosocial factors when the severely brain-damaged children were excluded. This kind of study has also been valuable in giving us information as to how symptoms at varying ages may disappear or develop into syndromes.

Retrospective Follow-Up Studies

Catch-Up Studies
The first well-controlled and also comprehensive retrospective catch-up study was the classic work of Robins (1974) in St. Louis. Robins recognized the value of 30-year-old records on children who had been seen and evaluated in a court-attached child guidance clinic, no longer in existence. She succeeded in tracing 90% of the 524 children, now adults. The majority of these children had had court appearances but some had shown evidence of neurotic problems or learning disabilities. (ADHD was not a diagnosis made at that time.) Robins also found 100 adults to serve as control subjects, whom she matched with the 524 probands. She found that most of the children who had been court referred had become adults with antisocial problems. Robins thus demonstrated that the methodology of assessing—through the use of structured interviews of adults—the psychiatric status of individuals who had been evaluated as children was feasible and provided us with invaluable information on the adult outcome of different childhood psychiatric disorders.

Another study using this methodology was the first controlled study of hyperactive children. Borland and Heckman (1966) selected boys from 25-year-old charts who they felt fitted a diagnosis of hyperactivity. Then they traced the adults and interviewed them; they also interviewed their brothers as normal control subjects. The use of siblings in this study may have skewed the results to minimize differences. Siblings of affected children have been found to have a minor form of many syndromes in child psychiatry.

There are many methodological difficulties with catch-up studies. The charts may have confusing or missing data. Standardized measurements may not have been available when the children were assessed. The diagnosis may have to be made as a probability from the available information in the chart. Two different researchers perusing a single chart may disagree on a diagnosis. Diagnostic criteria change over time, as do assessment techniques. Thus, diagnoses have to be assigned or reassigned from the available data. Finding the adults 25–30 years later may be difficult, and because the researcher has no rapport with the adults, they are more likely to refuse to come in.

These kinds of studies have been most successful when the childhood disorder was clearly delineated, such as in the case of antisocial acts that led to court referral.

Follow-Back Studies
Using this methodology of longitudinal studies, adults who have similar characteristics—for example, adoptees who are alcoholic (Goodwin et al. 1975) or a group of inpatient veterans with different current diagnoses (Gomez et al. 1981) or adults who have symptoms of ADHD (Wender et al. 1980)—are studied, and every attempt is made to trace back and clarify their childhood history. The difficulty with this technique is that it relies on the memory of the adults involved or on the memory of the now-grown-up children's parents. It is likely that a troubled adult's memories of childhood will be biased toward pathology. In spite of these limitations we have gained important information from follow-back studies. For example, such studies helped Wender et al. (1980) to recognize the adult form of attention deficit disorder (ADD) in childhood. In general, follow-back studies have indicated various childhood precursors of adult disorders, which may be different from the adult form of the disorder, such as in schizophrenia, or similar to the adult form of the disorder, such as in ADHD.

Prospective Follow-Up Studies
Although we shall discuss the methodological difficulties of prospective longitudinal studies in detail, including possible ways of overcoming these difficulties, this type of longitudinal study has

provided us with the most reliable information about the continuities and discontinuities of symptoms and the functional impairment of childhood psychopathological syndromes. It is only from prospective studies that we can see the course of individual development at predetermined regular time periods, which provides us with all the detailed information needed. Only prospective study of patients enables us to assess significant antecedent variables and the presence of risk factors, as well as how and when these operate. Prospective longitudinal studies have highlighted the frequency of comorbidity, and how this will affect outcome (August et al. 1983). These workers showed that the outcome for children with ADHD alone was significantly different from the outcome for children who had ADHD and conduct disorder. Dykman and Akerman's (1980) longitudinal study of 14-year-olds showed that children with learning disabilities had a good outcome unless the learning disabilities were associated with ADHD.

▼ Research Issues Related to Prospective Longitudinal Studies

Duration

The duration of a prospective longitudinal study is in itself a problem. The longer the study the more difficult it is to trace subjects who move out of town, or to motivate some subjects to continue to participate. The higher the loss of subjects the less reliable are the results, especially in view of Cox et al.'s (1977) findings that those lost to a study are likely to be the more impaired subjects. It is also harder to obtain funding for a long-term study. The researchers themselves (like their subjects) may move away, making continued follow-up more difficult, which is a factor of concern to granting agencies. The length of the study also necessitates that important intervening variables will occur that may influence outcome (illness, accident, jail, job loss, periods of recession to name only a few). The number of these variables are likely to be too large for most to be used as predictors of outcome.

Prospective longitudinal studies can range over a time period of 3–30 years. During that period a decision is made about the specific variables to be studied, the measures chosen to study these variables, and the frequency of assessment. It is wise to use more than one measure for a given variable, and to use structured interviews by unknown persons as well as nonstructured interviews by professionals whom the subjects trust. The more frequently assessments are made, such as once a year, the more information is obtained. However, the rate of refusal may increase if subjects are assessed too often and the study may become too difficult and expensive to carry out, the data too massive to handle.

Diagnostic Criteria

In our own study the diagnostic criteria changed from "hyperactive child" to DSM-II, DSM-III, DSM-III-R, and DSM-IV (American Psychiatric Association 1968, 1980, 1987, 1994), all of which have slightly different diagnostic criteria. This is a problem for all types of longitudinal studies. It is perhaps most easily manageable in the prospective study, in which more than one diagnostic system can be used. For example, when we looked, using several different diagnostic criteria, at how many of our children had had "conduct disorder," when they initially entered the study we found that very few had had this diagnosis.

Assessment Procedures and Validated Rating Scales

Different versions (e.g., initial and revised) of one scale may give different results. Some scales are useful for a given age period but not for another and have to be slightly or completely modified. If standardized scales exist for different age groups, it is difficult to know if a statistically significant change seen across the developmental years of the study in the probands represents a real change in that function or whether it is an artifact of the measurement. For example, our cohort of hyperactive children had lower results on the Wechsler Adult Intelligence Scale (WAIS) in adulthood than on the Wechsler Intelligence Scale for Children—Revised (WISC-R) in childhood. It was difficult to interpret this. Often, the same scale cannot be employed across the whole course of childhood, adolescence, and adulthood. When different scales are employed to measure the same function, it is hoped that they do indeed measure that same function.

Ethical Issues

The issue of informed consent should present little difficulty in longitudinal studies—compared, for example, with acute medication studies, in which unnecessary fear is sometimes introduced by informing the patient of every side effect of a medication ever noted. Our challenge was to try not to label our cohort over 15 years with a syndrome they might have more or less grown out of and often never remembered being told they had in the first place. We initially wanted to tell them we were following up on children who had had difficulties with paying attention. This was not acceptable to ethical review boards, which required the syndrome's name and character. Although we did use this full consent form, some of the children and parents resented or were upset about the diagnosis given 5 years later when they had forgotten what they had been told 5 years previously. Ian Murray (Weiss and Hechtman 1993), a subject in our follow-up study, described graphically in his chapter how he had felt "labeled" and how he had felt at times like a guinea pig, even though he acknowledged he had also benefited from partaking in the longitudinal study.

A similar problem occurred when we wanted to get employers' reports on probands and control subjects in their current job, during the 10- and 15-year follow-up when they were young adults. Research protocol demanded (as it should have) that we get not only verbal agreement but also written consent from our probands, for their employers to be contacted. None of them agreed to let their employer be contacted, and we did not blame them. In the end we composed a letter stating that we were "studying *normal young adults* with respect to their work performance. Would (the employer) kindly fill out an enclosed questionnaire on John Doe, currently employed at that company?" Although the probands loved this letter because it stressed normality, and all of them gave their consent, one employer wrote back, "If you think John Doe is a normal young adult, you have obviously never met him. . . ."

Control Group

Choice of Subjects
Children or adults who volunteer themselves as control subjects may have multiple motivations. For example, parents may have questions they want to ask a professional about their children, but are hesitant to make an appointment for this; or parents may be worried about their children, or the ways in which they are raising their children. Adolescents may have problems that they do not see as abnormal, but would like to discuss with a professional. In general, self-selection tends to sort out more troubled control subjects. In many studies control subjects are offered payment; this is often not enough to motivate them to come, and it may introduce bias. In our study we chose a child in the same classroom as the proband whose last name began with the same first or second letters (or closest to it). We then wrote to these children and strongly encouraged them to participate as control subjects. We agreed to see them to discuss this further and we offered to pay them in addition. Telling the parents of the control subjects their child had been chosen as a "normal child" to compare with troubled children was a bigger motivational bonus than the pay. Few refused, but the method of choice resulted in the normal control study being 1 year younger than the mean age of the probands. We eliminated the youngest children. We decided not to use sibling control subjects for reasons already outlined.

Matching One Group With Another
The most common variables on which matching is based in longitudinal studies are intelligence, socioeconomic class, age, and gender. Matching on the above variables is feasible for a study, yet it leaves out other very important variables on which one would theoretically wish to match: family functioning, criminality in a parent, child abuse, temporary placement in care, birth injury, comorbidity. Some of these factors could be used as exclusion factors. Other

more subtle aspects, such as the ability to make and keep friends, may be extremely important for final outcome but, as with likeability, are rarely matched for.

Exclusion and Inclusion Criteria

To select the cohort that will be followed, a decision has to be made about how to define inclusion criteria, and on what grounds to exclude a subject. In our study we excluded children with a WISC IQ under 85, children not currently living with their parents, and children with frank brain damage, epilepsy, or evidence of psychotic features. Other exclusion factors included child abuse, chaotic families, criminal parents, and temporary placement in care. Also, the exclusion criteria made criteria for ADHD selective, and also less generalizable, because many children with ADHD who had IQs slightly below 85 were ruled out. We now know the presence of comorbidity to be an exclusion criterion, although we had not sufficiently recognized this when we began the follow-up study. It was fortunate that our own inclusion criteria—which required the presence of problems with concentration, impulsivity, and restlessness—did exclude children with ADHD in whom conduct disorder was predominant (except in three cases). However, we did not exclude children with significant learning disabilities or oppositional traits. Diagnostic criteria for oppositional defiant disorder (DSM-III-R) were not available when we began our longitudinal study.

▼ Overcoming Duration Difficulties of Prospective Longitudinal Studies

Farrington (1991), in an important article on longitudinal research strategies, suggested that to overcome the problems related to the long duration of prospective studies, an accelerated longitudinal design could be utilized. In other words, to advance the knowledge about the development of criminal offenses and related psychopathology from birth to adulthood, Farrington advocated using several different cohorts for several years to cover the age span. An example would be following one cohort from birth to 6 years, a second cohort from 6 to 12 years, a third cohort from 12 to 18 years, and a fourth cohort from 18 to 24 years. All cohorts are regularly assessed over the same time period. This method not only reduces the time span of the study, but also reduces the changes that occur in subjects' environments over longer time periods, which may well affect their outcome. Examples of such changes are times of prosperity with high employment, times of recession with many lay-offs, changes in general prevalence of nonmedical drug use, changes in school curricula, and so on. The advantage of telescoping the time frame in this fashion is somewhat limited by not truly seeing the longitudinal course of the condition in the same individuals.

We can thus say categorically that without the information provided by longitudinal studies with their varying methodologies, our understanding of childhood syndromes of psychopathology would be severely limited, and incomplete.

In summary, longitudinal studies are of value in providing a view of adult outcome of childhood disorders, and how this outcome may be influenced by a variety of factors, such as life events, comorbidity, family functioning, and treatment. Furthermore, such studies often provide validation of the syndrome and strengthen the link between adult and child psychiatry. Finally, longitudinal studies may provide clues for more effective prevention and treatment.

▼ References

American Psychiatric Association: Diagnostic and Statistical Manual of Mental Disorders, 2nd Edition. Washington, DC, American Psychiatric Association, 1968

American Psychiatric Association: Diagnostic and Statistical Manual of Mental Disorders, 3rd Edition. Washington, DC, American Psychiatric Association, 1980

American Psychiatric Association: Diagnostic and Statistical Manual of Mental Disorders, 3rd Edition, Revised. Washington, DC, American Psychiatric Association, 1987

American Psychiatric Association: Diagnostic and Statistical Manual of Mental Disorders, 4th Edition. Washington, DC, American Psychiatric Association, 1994

August GI, Stewart MA, Holmes CS: A four year follow-up of hyperactive boys with and without conduct disorder. Br J Psychiatry 143:192–198, 1983

Biederman J, Faraone SY, Keenan K, et al: Evidence of familial association between attention deficit disorder and major affective disorders. Arch Gen Psychiatry 48:633–642, 1991

Borland BL, Heckman HK: Hyperactive boys and their brothers: a 25 year follow-up study. Arch Gen Psychiatry 33:669–675, 1966

Cox A, Rutter M, Yule B, et al: Bias resulting from missing information: some epidemiological findings. British Journal of Preventive Social Medicine 31:131–136, 1977

Dykman RA, Akerman P: Long Term Follow-Up Studies of Hyperactive Children in Advances in Behavioral Paediatrics, Vol 1. Greenwich, CT, JAL Press, 1980

Farrington DP: Longitudinal research strategies: advantages, problems and prospects. J Am Acad Child Adolesc Psychiatry 30: 369–391, 1991

Gittelman Klein R, Mannuzza S, Schenker R, et al: Hyperactive boys almost grown up: psychiatric status. Arch Gen Psychiatry 42:937–947, 1985

Gomez RL, Janowsky D, Zeitlin M, et al: Adult psychiatric diagnosis and symptoms compatible with the hyperactive child syndrome: a retrospective study. J Clin Psychiatry 42:389–394, 1981

Goodwin DW, Schutsinger F, Hermanson I, et al: Alcoholism and the hyperactive child syndrome. J Nerv Ment Dis 160:349–353, 1975

Laufer MW: Long term management and some follow-up findings on the use of drugs with minimal cerebral syndromes. Journal of Learning Disability 4:55–58, 1971

Laufer MW, Denhoff E: Hyperkinetic behaviour syndrome in children. Journal of Paediatrics 50:463–474, 1957

Robins LN: Deviant Children Grown Up: A Sociological and Psychiatric Study of Sociopathic Personality. Huntingdon, NY, RE Krieger, 1974

Rutter M: Longitudinal research: an empirical bias for the primary preventions of psychosocial disorders. Edited by Medinick SA, Baent AE. New York, Oxford University Press, 1985, pp 326–336

Shaffer D, Greenhill LA: A critical note on the validity of the hyperkinetic syndrome. Journal of Child Psychology 20:61–72,
1979

Szatmari P, Offord DR, Boyle MH: Ontario child health study: prevalence of attention deficit disorder with hyperactivity. J Child Psychol Psychiatry 30:219–230, 1989

Verhulst FC, Koot HM: Longitudinal research in child and adolescent
psychiatry. J Am Acad Child Adolesc Psychiatry 30:361–368,
1991

Weiss G, Hechtman L: Hyperactive Children Grown Up: ADHD in
Children, Adolescents, and Adults, 2nd Edition. New York, Guilford, 1993

Wender PH, Reimherr FW, Wood DR: Attention deficit disorder in
adults: a replication study of diagnosis and drug treatment. Arch
Gen Psychiatry 38:449–456, 1980

Werner EE: High risk children in young adulthood: a longitudinal
from birth to 32 years. Am J Orthopsychiatry 59:72–81, 1989

Chapter 2

Attention-Deficit/ Hyperactivity Disorder

Lily Hechtman, M.D., F.R.C.P.C.

In this chapter, I review the value and limitations of longitudinal research in child and adolescent psychiatry and how various methodological problems may account for the variability in different outcome studies. The adolescent and adult outcome for children who have attention-deficit/hyperactivity disorder (ADHD) is explored via a comprehensive review of various follow-up studies. In adolescence, about 70% of subjects still have ADHD and significant academic, social, and emotional problems. Children who also have aggression and/or conduct disorder generally have more negative outcome, and stimulant treatment does not appear to significantly affect this outcome.

This chapter is adapted from Hechtman L: "Long-Term Outcome in Attention-Deficit Hyperactivity Disorder." *Child and Adolescent Psychiatric Clinics of North America* 1:553–565, 1992. Used with permission.

In adulthood, generally the outcome is less negative, with some subjects functioning fairly well. However, many continue to have problems with concentration and impulsiveness. The resulting work and interpersonal difficulties are often accompanied by social and emotional problems. A small proportion of adults are seriously impaired psychiatrically and/or socially. Factors that may affect these various outcomes are discussed in this chapter.

In a recent review outlining the value and limitations of longitudinal research in child and adolescent psychiatry, Verhulst and Koot (1991) point out that longitudinal research is necessary

■ To assess which problems in children persist and which do not
■ To assess which early factors predict adult psychopathology
■ To evaluate the necessity and efficacy of treatment and prevention
■ To reveal causative mechanisms
■ To assess the validity of diagnostic constructs in terms of outcome.

However, studies on the long-term outcome of ADHD have given very diverse outcome pictures because of marked methodological differences of various outcome studies (Hechtman 1989; Weiss 1991).

▼ Methodological Problems

Prospective Versus Retrospective Follow-Up

Some outcome studies are prospective whereas others are retrospective. Retrospective studies can be *retrospective catch-up* (a diagnosis is made by reviewing old charts and then tracing the subjects), or *retrospective follow-back* (a group of adults with problems are evaluated regarding the presence of ADHD in their childhood). Because accurate diagnoses from sketchy old charts or skewed parental and patient memories are extremely difficult, only prospective studies are described.

Attrition Rate: Sample Size

Studies vary greatly in the proportion of the original sample that is lost to follow-up. Generally, the longer the follow-up period, the more subjects are lost. If the loss of subjects at follow-up becomes significant, the findings are questionable. It has been well documented by Cox et al. (1977) that subjects lost to follow-up often constitute a more pathological group. Even when attrition is not a problem, small sample size makes it difficult to assess statistical significance of the data obtained and gives one less confidence in the generalizability of the findings.

Diagnostic Criteria: Subject Characteristics

Follow-up studies often vary with regard to which diagnostic criteria are used. Subjects also may differ with regard to coexisting conditions such as learning disabilities or oppositional or conduct disorders. The coexistence of other conditions may significantly affect the picture at follow-up. In addition, subjects may vary on key factors such as intelligence (IQ), socioeconomic status (SES), severity and pervasiveness of symptoms, and type and amount of treatment received. Thus, the particular characteristics of the subject population may well affect long-term outcome.

Control Groups

Many follow-up studies do not have matched control or comparison groups whose members grew up at the same time as those in the study group. This deficiency prevents one from assessing if findings in the experimental group are significantly different from a matched normal control or comparison group and limits the utility of follow-up data.

Assessment Methods

Studies differ in how they assess follow-up subjects. Some researchers, such as Laufer (1971), use mailed questionnaires, whereas others, such as Hechtman and Weiss (1988), directly interview subjects and their families and obtain records from schools, employers, police, and courts.

The breadth of assessments also varies. Some studies look at one dimension, such as arrest records (Satterfield et al. 1982), whereas others carry out comprehensive assessments of psychiatric, academic, and social functioning (Weiss et al. 1985).

The assessment methods also vary with regard to whether standardized evaluations and forms are used and whether the evaluations are completed by subjects, parents, or professionals.

Age and Length of Follow-Up

Follow-up studies also differ in how old subjects are at follow-up and how long a follow-up period is involved. Thus, some studies have reported on latency-aged children with a 2-year follow-up (Riddle and Rapoport 1976), whereas others have reported on subjects 30 years of age in a 25-year follow-up (Borland and Heckman 1976).

The methodological difficulties and differences in these follow-up studies require that we evaluate them critically and draw conclusions with full awareness of their strengths and weaknesses.

The differences in these studies may account for the diverse findings and theories regarding long-term outcome of ADHD.

Cantwell (1985) succinctly summarized the differing theoretical views of ADHD outcome. An early theory advocated a developmental lag, which children outgrew in adolescence. A second theory suggested the continuation of symptoms into adulthood. A third theory postulated that ADHD may be a precursor to serious adult pathology. The critical review of recent studies of adolescent and adult outcome will illustrate which theory has the greatest empirical support and which factors may affect different outcomes.

▼ Outcome

In recent years, a number of review articles have addressed adolescent and adult outcome in ADHD (e.g., Hechtman 1985, 1989; Hechtman and Weiss 1983; Klein and Mannuzza 1991; Thorley 1984, 1988; Weiss 1985).

Adolescents

Only prospective controlled follow-up studies involving the ADHD adolescent-age group will be summarized here.

One of the earliest studies was conducted by Weiss et al. (1971). This comprehensive, 5-year prospective controlled follow-up study of 91 subjects ages 10–18 (mean 13.3 years) found that, compared with a control group matched for age, sex, IQ, and SES, adolescents with ADHD had poor self-esteem, more academic problems, and significant antisocial behavior; most also continued to be distractible, impulsive, and emotionally immature, although less hyperactive.

In another early study, Akerman et al. (1977) compared a normal control group ($N = 31$), a learning-disabled group ($N = 39$), and a third group whose members were learning disabled and hyperactive ($N = 23$). All subjects had IQs of at least 80 and were age 14 years at follow-up. The hyperactive learning-disabled group had significantly more oppositional or delinquent behavior and lower self-esteem. They were also more fidgety, impulsive, immature, and inattentive. Their academic performance was worse than that of the control group but not worse than that of the other learning-disabled group.

Satterfield et al. (1982) carried out a controlled prospective study of 110 hyperactive adolescents and 88 matched control subjects. At follow-up (mean age 17.3 years), 50% of the hyperactive subjects had had a felony arrest (for burglary, grand theft, or assault with a weapon) compared with less than 10% of the control subjects; 19% of the hyperactive subjects and none of the control subjects had been institutionalized. Neither SES nor stimulant treatment in childhood significantly influenced these results.

On a more optimistic note, Satterfield et al. (1981) reported on a 3-year prospective uncontrolled study of 100 hyperactive boys who received multimodal treatment. Treatment programs were individualized to the needs of each child and family, and included stimulant medication in addition to individual and/or group therapy for the child and parents. The group receiving longer treatment seemed to have better academic and social outcome.

Gittelman et al. (1985), in her prospective follow-up of 101 male adolescents, ages 16–23 years, compared these adolescents with 100 matched healthy control subjects and found that during early adolescence (between 13 and 15 years of age), 68% of the hyperactive subjects continued to meet diagnostic criteria for ADHD. This suggests that ADHD symptoms in adolescence remain fairly stable (Gittelman-Klein 1987).

Lambert et al. (1987) reassessed 59 pervasively hyperactive 12-year-old boys and 58 control subjects matched for age, race, and parental occupation. Information was obtained from parents, teachers, and children. Hyperactive subjects performed significantly worse than did control subjects on tests of IQ, academic achievement, cognitive development, and cognitive style, but *not* on tests of attention.

Hyperactive subjects also showed significantly more antisocial behavior as evidenced by increased school suspensions (14% vs. 2%), problems with law enforcement agencies (19% vs. 3%), and admission to juvenile facilities (5% vs. 0%).

Lambert et al.'s study concluded that 20% of the hyperactive subjects had no problems at follow-up. Some 37% had persistent learning, behavioral, or emotional problems, but were no longer receiving medical intervention (residual group). Another 43% of the hyperactive subjects were still being treated for hyperactivity and had learning, behavioral, or emotional difficulties (still hyperactive group). All hyperactive subjects received multiple treatments, which included pharmacological, educational, and psychological intervention.

The residual and still-hyperactive groups required more treatment. No early factors that might predict outcome could be identified. However, concurrent factors associated with the no-problem group included cognitive and behavioral maturity. The residual group showed cognitive immaturity but behavioral maturity, whereas the still-hyperactive group exhibited both cognitive and behavioral immaturity.

Cantwell and Baker (1989) did a 4-year follow-up of 151 children referred to a community speech and language clinic. Thirty-five children in this sample received an initial diagnosis of ADHD. Eighty percent of these subjects still had ADHD at follow-up. Five children had additional emotional disorders such as anxiety, affective, and obsessive-compulsive disorders. One child also had a conduct disorder, two had autism, and one had a transient tic disorder. Cantwell concluded that most children with ADHD continued to have the diagnosis at follow-up.

A series of articles by Barkley et al. (1990, 1991) and Fischer et al. (1990) describe an 8-year prospective comprehensive follow-up of 100 hyperactive subjects and 60 community control subjects. The average age at follow-up for the hyperactive and control-group subjects was about 15 years and 14 years, respectively. The authors reported that, at follow-up, 71.5% of the hyperactive subjects and 3% of the control-group subjects met DSM-III-R (American Psychiatric Association 1987) criteria for ADHD, whereas 60% of the hyperactive subjects and 11% of the control subjects also received the diagnosis of oppositional disorder. The presence of the oppositional disorder was associated with more negative mother/child interactions, greater ratings of home conflicts, and maternal psychological distress. In addition, about 40% of the hyperactive subjects and only 1.6% of the control-group subjects met criteria for conduct disorder. Conduct disorder was associated with greater use of cigarettes and marijuana (though not alcohol), and more school expulsions and suspensions.

Families of hyperactive subjects also tended to be less stable, with higher divorce rates, more frequent moves, and more frequent job changes. Fathers of hyperactive subjects also showed a greater incidence of antisocial behaviors.

Despite the availability and use of educational and mental health services (including medication), this outcome study indicates that most hyperactive subjects continue to have significant academic, social, and emotional problems in adolescence.

The importance for outcome of a comorbid diagnosis of conduct disorder has been pointed out by a number of researchers. Thus, August et al. (1983) followed a group of hyperactive subjects with and without conduct disorder and reassessed them at age 14 years. Subjects with both diagnoses continued to have symptoms of ADHD, but were also aggressive, noncompliant, antisocial, and used alcohol. The group that was only hyperactive at initial assessment had few conduct problems at follow-up. Thus, the importance of conduct disorder (rather than hyperactivity) in the development of antisocial behavior in adolescence is stressed.

The importance of the combined difficulties of attention deficit disorder (ADD) and delinquency on long-term outcome was also stressed by Moffitt (1990). In a large ($N = 435$) prospective follow-up of a male birth cohort from ages 3 to 15, the authors defined and compared four groups at age 13: a nondisordered group, a group that was only attention-deficit disordered, a group that was only delinquent, and a group that was both attention-deficit disordered *and* delinquent. Measures regarding antisocial behavior problems, verbal intelligence, reading difficulty, and family adversity were obtained every 2 years from ages 3 to 15. The ADD-positive delinquent group was consistently worse on measures of family adversity, verbal intelligence, and reading. Their antisocial behavior started before they were school age, increased when they entered school, and continued into adolescence. In contrast, the ADD-only boys had normal families, intelligence, and reading scores, and showed only mild antisocial behavior in middle childhood. Surprisingly, the delinquent-only boys showed no early problems with family ratings, intelligence, or reading and were relatively free of conduct problems until they initiated delinquency at age 13 years.

Generally, the review of the preceding articles suggests that some 70% of adolescents who had ADHD in childhood continue to have significant difficulties. Often they have symptoms that meet the diagnostic criteria for ADHD: restlessness, overactivity, and problems with attention and cognition. Subjects frequently have educational problems, with poor academic performance. Personality difficulties include immaturity and impulsivity, with social problems involving peers, teachers, and parents. Poor self-esteem is common. Antisocial behavior in adolescence is also frequent, particularly in children who also showed unsocialized aggression or conduct disorder when first referred.

Reviews by Hechtman (1985) and Thorley (1988) further suggest that stimulant treatment does not seem to have significantly affected the outcome outlined above.

Adults

A view of adult outcome of ADHD can be obtained from four different sources, including controlled prospective follow-up studies, retrospective studies, evidence of similar adult disorders, and family studies of children with ADHD.

Controlled Prospective Follow-Up Studies

For several reasons, the controlled prospective follow-up study provides the clearest, most reliable picture of adult outcome. First, the diagnosis is made by directly assessing the child and obtaining information from parents and teachers. Second, the hyperactive subjects and generally a matched control group are followed and periodically reassessed via standardized measures. Thus, prospective studies are not limited by sketchy old charts (as in retrospective studies) or selective patient and parental memories (as in adult patient or family studies). In addition, adults who are well but who were affected in childhood are also seen, thereby providing a more comprehensive and less negatively biased picture. Unfortunately, to date, few controlled prospective follow-up studies have followed hyperactive subjects into adulthood.

Weiss and Hechtman (1993) carried out a controlled prospective follow-up study in which 104 children were initially assessed when they were age 6–12 years. Ninety-one were reassessed at the mean age of 13.3 in a 5-year follow-up; 75 were seen again at the mean age of 19 in a 10-year follow-up; and 64 were seen at the mean age of 25 in a 15-year follow-up. In adolescence, a control group matching the hyperactive subjects in age, sex, IQ, and SES was selected and followed with the hyperactive group. Half of the subjects lost to follow-up could not be traced and probably constituted a somewhat negative outcome group. The other half, who were contacted by telephone, gave a detailed response indicating that they were doing well but did not wish to come in to be reevaluated and be reminded of past problems. They reflected a more positive outcome group. The comprehensive assessments included demographic, academic, work, psychiatry, and social (including antisocial behavior and drug and alcohol abuse), as well as physiological and psychological parameters. Data were obtained via direct interviews with subjects and parents and reports from schools, employers, and the court system.

Generally, the hyperactive subjects fared worse than the matched control group. Demographically, they moved more frequently with fewer hyperactive subjects living at home. Academically (Weiss et al. 1985), the hyperactive individuals had completed less education, had failed more grades, and had obtained lower marks. They also continued to do worse on various cognitive tests (Hopkins et al. 1979). In the realm of work (Weiss et al. 1978), most hyperactive subjects were gainfully employed but their work status was generally inferior to that of control subjects, and they changed jobs more frequently. Hyperactive adults had more court referrals and more nonmedical drug use (Hechtman et al. 1984a; Hechtman and Weiss 1988). Twenty-three percent of the hyperactive subjects and only 2.4% of control subjects met DSM-III (American Psychiatric Association 1980) criteria for antisocial personality disorder.

Recently, Herrero et al. (1994) conducted a comprehensive chart review of these same hyperactive subjects who were followed prospectively for 15 years at 5-year intervals. They identified four subgroups in the developmental course of antisocial behavior in adulthood: those who never presented with antisocial problems (26%); those with continuing antisocial problems from childhood to adulthood (30%); those who showed initial antisocial behavior that did not continue (18%); and those who exhibited antisocial behavior initially and/or in adolescence but not in adulthood (26%). The group with continuing antisocial behavior from childhood to adulthood also had the most subjects with continuing hyperactive symptoms (70%) and other psychiatric diagnoses (90%). By contrast, subjects in the other groups who had continuing symptoms of the hyperactive syndrome ranged from 18% to 33%. Generally, girls were more likely to be in the first group that never presented with any antisocial behavior. Thus, ADHD was a risk factor for antisocial outcome in boys but not in girls. The absence of behavior-related problems at initial intake was a predictive factor for the absence of antisocial disorders in adulthood; however, the presence of such initial problems is not predictive of an antisocial outcome. Where such initial problems did not result in adult antisocial outcome, it was found that mental health of family members may have acted as a protective factor.

In addition to the antisocial problems outlined above, two-thirds of the hyperactive group were troubled by at least one disabling core symptom of the syndrome: restlessness, impulsivity, and/or problems with sustained attention. Hyperactive subjects also made more suicide attempts (Weiss et al. 1985) and had poorer social skills and

self-esteem (Hechtman et al. 1980). Generally, the hyperactive subjects presented with more symptoms and received more psychiatric
diagnoses.

Physiological measures showed no differences in height, weight,
blood pressure, pulse (Hechtman et al. 1978b), or electroencepha-
logram (EEG) (Hechtman et al. 1978a). A comparison of EEGs of
hyperactive subjects over time (initially, 5- and 10-year follow-up)
indicated that normalization of EEGs tended to take place in adolescence.

Gittelman et al. (1985) conducted a similar comprehensive controlled follow-up study of 101 hyperactive subjects and 100
matched normal control subjects. The age range was 16–23 years
with a mean age of 18 years. Ninety-eight percent were found at 5-
to 11-year follow-up (mean 9 years). Results indicated that 31% of
the hyperactive subjects versus 3% of the control subjects met DSM-
III criteria for a full ADHD syndrome. Twenty-seven percent of
hyperactive adults versus 8% of control subjects had either conduct
or antisocial personality disorder, and 16% of the hyperactive adults
versus 3% of the control subjects had drug use disorder (other than
alcohol). Other conditions such as affective or anxiety disorders did
not differ significantly between the two groups. It also seems that
the likelihood of developing conduct disorder is greater if ADHD
persists and that substance abuse is often linked to or follows the
conduct disorder. This study suggests that hyperactive individuals
are more prone to having ADHD, antisocial personality disorders,
and substance abuse disorders in adulthood and that these three
conditions aggregate in the same individuals.

The importance of this comorbidity is seen in the study of Mannuzza et al. (1989), who looked at New York state judicial records
of previously hyperactive boys and control subjects (ages 17–24,
mean age 22). The hyperactive boys were arrested twice as often as
the control subjects (39% vs. 20%, $P < .01$), and were more likely
to have been charged with an aggressive or felonious offense. More
hyperactive boys were convicted and incarcerated (9% vs. 1%, $P <$
.02). In addition, more of the hyperactive boys had multiple arrests
(23% vs. 8%, $P < .001$) and multiple convictions (18% vs. 2%,
$P < .001$).

A diagnosis of antisocial personality disorder at follow-up was a strong predictor of arrests, but the presence of ADHD (without antisocial disorder) was not. Thus, this study did not support a straightforward link between hyperactivity and criminality or arrests, but suggested the necessary presence of an antisocial personality disorder diagnosis. However, it is unclear if childhood ADHD increases the risk of developing antisocial personality disorder and criminality in adulthood without the presence of childhood conduct disorder.

In a companion article involving the same follow-up subjects, Mannuzza et al. (1988) showed that hyperactive individuals who received no DSM-III diagnosis at follow-up did worse than control subjects in school adjustment, but no differences were seen in occupational adjustment, temperament, alcohol use, or antisocial behavior. Thus, one can see that some hyperactive subjects have positive outcomes whereas others do not. Continuation of ADHD symptoms and the development of antisocial personality disorder seem key in determining this diverse outcome.

A 17-year follow-up of the same subjects, 24–33 years of age (mean age 26) (Mannuzza et al. 1993) suggests that there is an overall reduction in rates of dysfunction in adulthood, although the pattern of outcome is similar to that found at age 18 years. Thus, at mean age 26 years, 11% of hyperactive subjects versus 1% of control subjects ($P < .06$) had ADHD. Eighteen percent of hyperactive subjects vs. 2% of control subjects ($P < .001$) had antisocial personality disorder, and 16% of hyperactive subjects versus 4% of control subjects ($P < .02$) had substance use disorder (other than alcohol). Again, there was no increased risk for other conditions, such as affective or anxiety disorder in the hyperactive group.

Loney et al. (1983) compared 22 hyperactive adults, ages 21–23, with their brothers. The hyperactive adults were diagnosed more frequently (45% vs. 18%) as having an antisocial personality disorder, but did not have more drug or alcohol use disorder when compared with their brothers. Even though they reported no increased contact with police, the hyperactive adults were incarcerated more frequently than their brothers (41% vs. 5%, $P < .02$), suggesting that they had more serious offenses, particularly against other persons. Loney's results are thus similar to other studies of adult outcome.

Many authors (August et al. 1983; Barkley et al. 1990, 1991; Gittelman et al. 1985; Moffitt 1990; Mannuzza et al. 1989) have stressed the importance of the coexistence between hyperactivity or ADHD and conduct or antisocial personality disorder in determining poor adult outcome as opposed to hyperactivity alone. However, Farrington (1990) followed 411 inner city London boys from ages 8 to 30. In childhood, the boys were classified as to whether they had hyperactivity, impulsivity, and attentional problems (HIA), as well as conduct and oppositional disorder. Subjects were thus divided into four groups: those having HIA *and* conduct problems ($n = 59$), those having only HIA and no conduct disorder problems ($n = 34$), those having no HIA and only conduct disorder problems ($n = 40$), and, finally, those having neither HIA nor conduct disorder problems ($n = 278$). Not surprisingly, the group with HIA *and* conduct disorder problems had the worst prognosis, with chronic criminal behavior. However, the group that had only HIA and no conduct disorder problems in childhood also had some later criminal behavior. This finding is somewhat surprising because it suggests that hyperactivity alone may have increased risk for later criminality. However, the results of this study are different from the other studies outlined above, which suggest the importance of the coexistence between ADHD and conduct disorder in negative adult outcome and not hyperactivity alone. This area remains unclear and controversial and requires further investigation.

Retrospective Studies

A number of previous reviews dealing with adolescent and adult outcome of children with ADHD described retrospective outcome studies in some detail (Hechtman 1989; Hechtman and Weiss 1983; Thorley 1984; Weiss 1985). To illustrate the general nature of such studies and the type of outcomes they report, two studies will be briefly described.

Borland and Heckman (1976) compared 20 men (average age 30 years) whose childhood medical records conformed to diagnostic criteria for hyperactive child syndrome with their brothers (mean age 26 years). The hyperactive men generally had completed high school and were steadily employed and self-supporting. However, compared with their brothers, they had more work and emotional problems.

Feldman et al. (1979) conducted a 10- to 12-year retrospective follow-up study on 48 young adults (mean age 21 years) who had previously been diagnosed as hyperactive. Almost all of the hyperactive individuals (91%) were either in school or working. However, compared with their siblings, the hyperactive subjects had lower educational achievement, poor self-esteem, and more problems with drug and alcohol use.

Evidence of Similar Adult Disorders

Another view of adult outcome of ADHD is derived from adult patients whose symptoms resemble those found in ADHD. Gaultieri et al. (1985), Mattes et al. (1984), Wender et al. (1981), and Wood et al. (1976) have all described studies involving such adult patients. Some of these patients have childhood histories consistent with the condition and others do not. Some of these patients seem to benefit from stimulant medication, whereas for others such medication has no positive effect. Factors that determine this adult responsiveness are unclear, as is the whole question of whether these adults in fact portray adult outcome of childhood ADHD.

Family Studies of Children With ADHD

Family studies of children with ADHD presuppose that by examining the adult relatives of children with ADHD, one gets some view of adult outcome of this condition. Some of these studies are comprehensively reviewed by Weiss and Hechtman (1993) in Chapter 12 of their book.

Generally, early family studies by Morrison (1980), Morrison and Stewart (1971, 1973), Stewart and Morrison (1980), and Cantwell (1972) suggest that biological parents of hyperactive children have a higher prevalence of sociopathy, hysteria, and alcoholism compared with parents of normal control subjects. The authors also felt that significantly more parents of hyperactive children had themselves been hyperactive as children. This increased pathology was not seen in adoptive parents of hyperactive children.

In comparing families of hyperactive children with families of children with other psychiatric diagnoses, Morrison (1980) found the parents of the hyperactive children had significantly more antisocial personality disorder and Briquet's syndrome (hysteria).

Parents of the children in the comparison group had other diagnoses (e.g., endogenous psychosis). However, the two groups of parents did not differ in the level of alcoholism.

Stewart and Morrison (1980) also found a higher incidence of unipolar but not bipolar affective disorder in combined second-degree blood relatives of hyperactive children.

Early family studies did not clearly distinguish between purely hyperactive children and those who had hyperactivity or ADHD combined with conduct disorder and/or oppositional disorder. Recent studies that look at this comorbidity suggest that children with these combined diagnoses may have significantly different family patterns than children who have only ADHD.

Biederman et al. (1987) evaluated first-degree relatives of 22 children with ADHD and 29 normal control subjects. Fourteen (64%) of the ADHD children also had the diagnosis of conduct or oppositional disorder. Relatives of this group of children had significantly more antisocial disorder, oppositional disorder, antisocial personality disorder, nonbipolar depressive disorder, and overanxious disorder, compared with relatives of normal control subjects and hyperactive children without coexisting conduct or oppositional disorder. Relatives of ADHD children with and without conduct or oppositional disorder did not differ in their high rates of ADHD (34%, respectively). This was significantly higher than the rate of ADHD in relatives of normal control subjects. Interestingly, the incidence of drug and alcohol abuse and dependence did not differ significantly in the three groups.

Lahey et al. (1988) also compared parental pathology in children (6–13 years of age) with conduct disorder ($n = 37$), with ADHD ($n = 18$), and with both disorders. Parents of children with conduct disorder were more likely to abuse substances. Mothers of children with conduct disorders were more often depressed and more frequently had the triad of antisocial personality disorder, substance abuse, and somatization disorder. In contrast, parents of children with ADHD only did not have any significant disorder. However, fathers of children with both conduct disorder *and* ADHD were more likely to have a history of aggression, arrest, and imprisonment.

Barkley et al. (1990), in their 8-year follow-up of hyperactive children, also collected information on the biological fathers of these children. They found that fathers of hyperactive children compared with fathers of normal control-group children had a history of significantly more antisocial acts, alcohol abuse, police contacts, and arrests. Their job histories were less stable, and they were generally less financially responsible. The authors concluded that 11% of fathers of hyperactive children met DSM-III-R criteria for antisocial personality disorder as opposed to 1.6% of fathers of normal control-group children ($P < .05$). When the authors examined the antisocial acts of fathers of children with hyperactivity, with and without associated conduct disorder, they found that the fathers of children with hyperactivity *and* conduct disorder had more antisocial acts than those with hyperactivity alone. However, fathers of children who were only hyperactive still had more antisocial acts than fathers of normal control-group children.

These studies clearly suggest that the combination of ADHD and conduct disorder is associated with significant parental pathology. The possible connections between parental pathology, childhood ADHD, and its adult outcome were explored in a study by Cadoret and Stewart (1991). The authors studied 283 adoptees ages 18–40 years. The adoptees were divided into two groups based on whether biological parents showed evidence (from adoption agency records) of psychiatric problems or behavioral disturbance. In addition to evaluation of biological parents from agency records, direct evaluation of adoptees and adoptive parents was also carried out.

The authors found that criminality or delinquency on the part of biological parents predicted increased antisocial personality disorder in adult adoptees *only* when the adoptee had been placed in a lower SES home. The lower SES home had no effect on development of adult antisocial personality disorder when there was no criminality in the biological background.

The importance of the environmental factors was also seen in the fact that psychiatric problems in the adoptive home were associated with aggressivity syndrome, and lower SES of the adoptive home increased the incidence of ADHD syndrome.

Aggressivity but *not* ADHD predicted antisocial personality disorder in adult adoptees.

This study demonstrates the importance of genetic (biological parental pathology) *and* environmental (SES and pathology of adoptive family) factors in the development of adult antisocial personality disorder.

The adult outcome of ADHD disorder may thus be influenced by the interaction of a number of factors: the continuation of the syndrome, the coexistence of other conditions (e.g., conduct and/or oppositional disorder), SES, and parental pathology. It will become the challenge of future research to clarify the impact of these factors on outcome and to develop interventions that will adequately address these problems and result in more positive adult outcome.

▼ Summary

As seen in this review of various types of follow-up studies, the adult outcome of children with ADHD can vary significantly (Hechtman et al. 1981). Generally, three different outcome groups can be detected. The first group is composed of ADHD subjects who in adulthood function fairly well and not significantly differently from a matched normal control group. A second group is composed of adults who continue to have significant problems with concentration, impulsiveness, and social and emotional functioning. These symptoms often result in difficulties with work, interpersonal relationships, poor self-esteem, impulsivity, irritability, anxiety, and emotional lability. The vast majority of young adults who are hyperactive fall into this group. Finally, a third group includes hyperactive individuals with significant psychiatric and/or antisocial pathology. These hyperactive adults may be seriously depressed, even suicidal, or may be heavily involved in drug or alcohol abuse or significant antisocial behavior (e.g., assault, armed robbery, breaking and entering, or drug dealing). This negative adult outcome is seen in a relatively small proportion of hyperactive children.

Factors that are associated with positive or negative outcome were explored by Hechtman et al. (1984b), Loney et al. (1983), and Mannuzza et al. (1990). Generally, one is left with the impression that adult outcome is not associated with a particular initial variable, but with the additive interaction of personality characteristics, and social, familial, and environmental parameters. However, some variables may prove particularly important. These include mental health of family members, IQ, and SES. Recent studies also implicate the importance of continuation of the ADHD symptoms (Gittelman et al. 1985) and the coexistence of significant aggression and conduct disorder (August et al. 1983; Barkley et al. 1990; Cadoret and Stewart 1991) in influencing adult outcome.

We are left with the challenge of unraveling how these factors interact and how they influence outcome, and what interventions are needed to ensure a more positive adult outcome.

▼ References

Akerman P, Dykman R, Peters J: Teenage status of hyperactive and nonhyperactive learning disabled boys. Am J Orthopsychiatry 47:577–596, 1977

American Psychiatric Association: Diagnostic and Statistical Manual of Mental Disorders, 3rd Edition. Washington, DC, American Psychiatric Association, 1980

American Psychiatric Association: Diagnostic and Statistical Manual of Mental Disorders, 3rd Edition, Revised. Washington, DC, American Psychiatric Association, 1987

August GJ, Steward MA, Holmes CS: A four year follow-up of hyperactive boys with and without conduct disorder. Br J Psychiatry 143:192–198, 1983

Barkley RA, Fischer M, Edelbrock CS, et al: The adolescent outcome of hyperactive children diagnosed by research criteria: an 8 year prospective follow-up study. J Am Acad Child Adolesc Psychiatry 29:546–557, 1990

Barkley RA, Fischer M, Edelbrock CS, et al: The adolescent outcome of hyperactive children diagnosed by research criteria, III: mother-child interactions, family conflicts and maternal psychopathology. J Child Psychol Psychiatry 32:233–255, 1991

Biederman J, Munik K, Knee D: Conduct and oppositional disorders in clinically referred children with attention deficit disorder: a controlled family study. J Am Acad Child Adolesc Psychiatry 26:724–727, 1987

Borland B, Heckman H: Hyperactive boys and their brothers: a 25 year follow-up study. Arch Gen Psychiatry 33:669–676, 1976

Cadoret JR, Stewart MA: An adoption study of attention deficit hyperactivity/aggression and their relationship to adult antisocial personality. Compr Psychiatry 32:73–82, 1991

Cantwell D: Psychiatric illness in families of hyperactive children. Arch Gen Psychiatry 27:414–423, 1972

Cantwell D: Hyperactive children have grown up: what have we been learning about what happens to them. Arch Gen Psychiatry 42:102–108, 1985

Cantwell D, Baker L: Stability and natural history of DSM-III childhood diagnoses. J Am Acad Child Adolesc Psychiatry 28:691–700, 1989

Cox A, Rutter M, Yule B: Bias resulting from missing information: some epidemiological findings. British Journal of Preventive and Social Medicine 31:131–136, 1977

Farrington DP: Long term criminal outcomes of hyperactivity-impulsivity-attention deficit (HIA) and conduct problems in childhood, in Straight and Devious Pathways From Childhood to Adulthood. Edited by Robins LN, Rutter M. New York, Cambridge University Press, 1990, pp 62–82

Feldman S, Denhoff E, Denhoff J: The attention disorders and related syndromes outcome in adolescence and young adult life, in Minimal Brain Dysfunction: A Developmental Approach. Edited by Denhoff E, Stern L. New York, Musson Publishers, 1979, pp 133–148

Fischer M, Barkley RA, Edelbrock CS, et al: The adolescent outcome of hyperactive children diagnosed by research criteria, II: academic, attentional and neuropsychological states. J Consult Clin Psychol 58:580–588, 1990

Gaultieri C, Ondrusek M, Finley C: Attention deficit disorder in adults. Clin Neuropharmacol 8:345–356, 1985

Gittelman-Klein R: Prognosis of attention deficit disorder and its management. Adolescent Pediatrics in Review 8:216–223, 1987

Gittelman R, Mannuzza S, Shenker R, et al: Hyperactive boys almost grown-up. Arch Gen Psychiatry 42:937–947, 1985

Hechtman L: Adolescent outcome of hyperactive children treated with stimulants in childhood: a review. Psychopharmacol Bull 21:178–191, 1985

Hechtman L: Attention deficit hyperactivity disorder in adolescence and adulthood: an updated follow-up. Psychiatric Annals 19: 597–603, 1989

Hechtman L, Weiss G: Long-term outcome of hyperactive children. Am J Orthopsychiatry 53:532–541, 1983

Hechtman L, Weiss G: Controlled prospective 15-year follow-up of hyperactives as adults: non-medical drug and alcohol use and antisocial behaviour. Can J Psychiatry 31:557–567, 1988

Hechtman L, Weiss G, Metrakos K: Hyperactives as young adults: current and longitudinal electroencephalographic evaluation and its relation to outcome. Can Med Assoc J 118:912–923, 1978a

Hechtman L, Weiss G, Perlman T: Growth and cardiovascular measures in hyperactive individuals as young adults and in matched normal controls. Can Med Assoc J 118:1247–1250, 1978b

Hechtman L, Weiss G, Perlman T: Hyperactives as young adults: self-esteem and social skills. Can J Psychiatry 25:478–483, 1980

Hechtman L, Weiss G, Perlman T, et al: Hyperactives as young adults: various clinical outcomes. Adolesc Psychiatry 9:295–306, 1981

Hechtman L, Weiss G, Perlman T, et al: Hyperactives as young adults: past and current antisocial behavior (stealing, drug abuse) and moral development. Am J Orthopsychiatry 54:415–425, 1984a

Hechtman L, Weiss G, Perlman T, et al: Hyperactives as young adults: initial predictors of adult outcome. J Am Acad Child Psychiatry 25:250–260, 1984b

Herrero ME, Hechtman L, Weiss G: Antisocial disorders in hyperactive subjects from childhood to adulthood: predictive factors and characteristics of subgroups. Am J Orthopsychiatry 64:510–521, 1994

Hopkins J, Perlman T, Hechtman L, et al: Cognitive style in adults originally diagnosed as hyperactives. J Child Psychol Psychiatry 20:209–216, 1979

Klein RG, Mannuzza S: Long-term outcome of hyperactive children: a review. J Am Acad Child Adolesc Psychiatry 30:383–387, 1991

Lahey B, Piacentini J, McBurnett M, et al: Psychopathology in the parents of children with conduct disorder and hyperactivity. J Am Acad Child Adolesc Psychiatry 27:163–170, 1988

Lambert N, Hartsaugh C, Sassone D: Persistence of hyperactivity symptoms from childhood to adolescence. Am J Orthopsychiatry 57:22–31, 1987

Laufer M: Long-term management and some follow-up findings on the use of drugs with minimal cerebral syndromes. Journal of Learning Disabilities 4:55–58, 1971

Loney J, Whaley-Klahn MA, Kosier T, et al: Hyperactive boys and their brothers at 21: predictors of aggressive and antisocial outcomes, in Prospective Studies of Crime and Delinquency. Edited by Van Dusen KT, Mednick SA. Boston, MA, Kluwer-Nijhoff, 1983, pp 181–206

Mannuzza S, Gittelman-Klein R, Bonagura N: Hyperactive boys almost grown up, II: status of subjects without a mental disorder. Arch Gen Psychiatry 45:13–18, 1988

Mannuzza S, Gittelman-Klein R, Horowitz-Konig P, et al: Hyperactive boys almost grown-up, IV: criminality and its relationship to psychiatric status. Arch Gen Psychiatry 46:1073–1079, 1989

Mannuzza S, Klein RG, Konig PH, et al: Childhood predictors of psychiatric status in the young adulthood of hyperactive boys: a study controlling for chance associations, in Straight and Devious Pathways From Childhood to Adulthood. New York, Cambridge University Press, 1990, pp 279–299

Mannuzza S, Klein RG, Bessler A, et al: Adult outcome of hyperactive boys. Arch Gen Psychiatry 50:565–576, 1993

Mattes J, Boswell L, Oliver H: Methylphenidate effects on symptoms of attention deficit disorder in adults. Arch Gen Psychiatry 41:1059–1063, 1984

Moffitt TE: Juvenile delinquency and attention deficit disorder: boys' developmental trajectories from age 3 to age 15. Child Dev 61:893–910, 1990

Morrison J: Adult psychiatric disorders in parents of hyperactive children. Am J Psychiatry 137:825–827, 1980

Morrison J, Stewart M: A family study of the hyperactive child syndrome. Biol Psychiatry 3:189–195, 1971

Morrison J, Stewart M: The psychiatric status of legal families of adopted hyperactives. Arch Gen Psychiatry 28:888–891, 1973

Riddle K, Rapoport J: A two-year follow-up of 72 hyperactive boys. J Nerv Ment Dis 162:126–134, 1976

Satterfield J, Satterfield B, Cantwell D: Three year multimodality treatment study of 100 hyperactive boys. J Pediatr 98:680–688, 1981

Satterfield J, Hoppe C, Schell A: Prospective study of delinquency in 110 adolescent boys with attention deficit disorder and 88 normal adolescent boys. Am J Psychiatry 139:797–798, 1982

Stewart M, Morrison J: Affective disorders among the relatives of hyperactive children. J Child Psychol Psychiatry 14:209–212, 1973

Thorley G: Review of follow-up and follow-back studies of childhood hyperactivity. Psychol Bull 96:116–132, 1984

Thorley G: Adolescent outcome for hyperactive children. Arch Dis Child 63:1181–1183, 1988

Verhulst FC, Koot HM: Longitudinal research in child and adolescent psychiatry. J Am Acad Child Adolesc Psychiatry 30:361–368, 1991

Weiss G: Follow up studies on outcome of hyperactive children. Psychopharmacol Bull 21:169–177, 1985

Weiss G: Attention deficit hyperactivity disorder, in Child and Adolescent Psychiatry: A Comprehensive Textbook. Edited by Lewis M. Baltimore, MD, Williams & Wilkins, 1991, pp 544–611

Weiss G, Hechtman L: Hyperactive Children Grown Up, 2nd Edition. New York, Guilford, 1993

Weiss G, Minde K, Werry J, et al: A five year follow-up study of 91 hyperactive school children. Arch Gen Psychiatry 24:409–414, 1971

Weiss G, Hechtman L, Perlman T: Hyperactives as young adults: school, employers and self-rating scales obtained during 10 year follow-up evaluation. Am J Orthopsychiatry 48:438–445, 1978

Weiss G, Hechtman L, Perlman T, et al: Hyperactives in young adulthood: a controlled prospective ten-year follow-up of 75 children. Arch Gen Psychiatry 36:675–681, 1979

Weiss G, Hechtman L, Milroy T, et al: Psychiatric status of hyperactives as adults: a controlled prospective 15-year follow-up of 63 hyperactive children. J Am Acad Child Psychiatry 23:211–220, 1985

Wender P, Reimher F, Wood D: Attention deficit disorder in adults. Arch Gen Psychiatry 38:449–456, 1981

Wood D, Reimher F, Wender P, et al: Diagnosis and treatment of MBD in adults. Arch Gen Psychiatry 33:1453–1460, 1976

Comorbidity in Outcome of Attention-Deficit/ Hyperactivity Disorder

**Joseph Biederman, M.D.,
Stephen V. Faraone, Ph.D., and
Kathleen Kiely, B.A.**

The long-term outcome of childhood psychopathology has been a major concern of clinicians, researchers, patients, and families. As
other chapters in this book show, longitudinal
research has provided a valuable source of empirical answers to the many questions about
long-term outcome. In this chapter, we highlight a key issue that complicates studies of
outcome and their interpretation: psychiatric
comorbidity. Although childhood psychiatric

This work was supported, in part, by USPHS (NIMH)
grant RO1 MH41314-01A2 and grant R01 MH50657-01
(J.B.).

disorders were originally defined as discrete, nonoverlapping entities, a growing clinical and epidemiological literature shows that this is not the case (Achenbach 1993; Angold and Costello 1993; Biederman et al. 1991a, 1992; Caron and Rutter 1991). This work shows that having one psychiatric disorder places children at risk for having another. We address the issue of psychiatric comorbidity by examining studies of children, adolescents, and adults with attention-deficit/hyperactivity disorder (ADHD), because of its extensive comorbidity with other disorders. However, the issue of comorbidity is a general one that cannot be ignored in the implementation and interpretation of long-term outcome studies.

When used descriptively, the term *comorbidity* refers to the presence of two or more disorders in the same child. However, the term is often used to indicate that two disorders occur together more often than expected by chance. When used in the latter fashion, we can distinguish between true and artifactual comorbidity.

Caron and Rutter (1991) list six sources of artifactual comorbidity. The most well-known of these is Berkson's bias (also called referral bias). This refers to the fact that children who are referred to treatment are more likely to have multiple disorders compared with nonreferred children. This is intuitively sensible. For example, among all children with separation anxiety disorder, those who are also depressed are more likely to be referred to clinics than those who are not. Thus, children with two disorders may be overrepresented in clinic and hospital populations. Selection biases can also occur in epidemiological studies if children are screened before selection. If the screening method uses a broad-band measure of psychopathology, then children with more than one disorder will be overrepresented in the samples.

Caron and Rutter also describe several nosological factors that can lead to spurious comorbidity. First, they note that the concept of comorbidity relies on a categorical approach to psychiatric nosology. If disorders are conceived of as extreme levels of traits or dimensions, then the concept of comorbidity is no longer relevant. Instead, one would assess the degree to which dimensional traits were correlated with one another.

Another nosological issue is the problem of overlapping diagnostic criteria. For example, the diagnostic criteria for both ADHD and major depression include difficulty concentrating. Because ADHD symptoms tend to be chronic, children with ADHD will more easily attain the diagnosis of depression because, regardless of whether they have depression, many of them will already have one of its symptoms.

Caron and Rutter's last three sources of artifactual comorbidity occur because the diagnostic taxonomy is simply wrong. This occurs when disorders are too finely subdivided, when one disorder is a prodrome of another, or when one disorder is a manifestation of another. As Achenbach (1993) points out, when substantial comorbidity is discovered, we should consider reassessing the validity of the comorbid psychiatric diagnoses.

Although artifactual causes of comorbidity cannot be ignored, we must also consider the possibility that comorbidity indicates etiological relationships between disorders. Caron and Rutter (1991) outline four possibilities. First, two disorders may share risk factors. For example, if psychosocial stress causes both anxiety and depression, then we would expect the two disorders to occur together more often than would be expected by chance. Second, although the risk factors for two disorders may be distinct, they may be correlated with each other. If low social class is a risk factor for one disorder and malnutrition a risk factor for another, then the two disorders will co-occur due to the association between social class and nutrition.

Third, it is possible that the comorbid condition is a meaningful syndrome that is nosologically distinct from the two disorders that constitute it. For example, Faraone et al. (1991b) present family genetic data suggesting that the combination of ADHD and conduct disorder may be etiologically distinct from each disorder by itself. Finally, it is possible that one disorder increases the risk for the other. For example, children with conduct disorder are more likely to be exposed to alcohol and illicit drugs. Thus, comorbidity between conduct and substance use disorders could reflect differences in environmental exposure between children with conduct disorders and other children. Moreover, as Angold and Costello (1993) note, it is possible that one disorder causes the other. For example, in some cases, depressive or anxiety disorders may cause alcohol abuse (i.e., through use for self-medication of symptoms).

Biederman et al. (1987a, 1991a, 1991b, 1992) and Faraone et al. (1993a) have proposed a hypothesis-testing framework that uses

family genetic data to determine the substantive causes of psychiatric comorbidity. Their approach is based in part on models developed by Leckman et al. (1983), Pauls et al.(1986a, 1986b), and
Reich et al. (1972, 1979). In stating these hypotheses, the expected
differences are relative to normal control groups.

According to the first hypothesis, if ADHD and the comorbid
disorder are etiologically independent, we would expect to find high
rates of ADHD in relatives of both children with ADHD and those
with ADHD plus the comorbid disorder, but an increased rate of
the comorbid disorder only among relatives of the ADHD plus comorbidity subgroup. The second hypothesis states that if ADHD
and the comorbid disorder share common familial etiological factors, we would expect to find high rates of ADHD and the comorbid
disorder in relatives of both subjects with ADHD and subjects with
ADHD plus the comorbid disorder compared with relatives of normal control subjects. Finally, the third hypothesis states that if
ADHD plus the comorbid disorder is a distinct familial subtype, we
would expect to find high rates of ADHD in relatives of both children with ADHD and those with ADHD plus the comorbid disorder
compared with relatives of normal control subjects, but high rates
of the comorbid disorder only in relatives of children with ADHD
plus the comorbid disorder. In addition, ADHD and the comorbid
disorder should cosegregate in these families. We use the term
cosegregate to indicate that the disorders are transmitted together,
not independently. In other words, the degree of comorbidity in the
relatives is greater than what would be expected by chance.

▼ Comorbidity in Children and Adolescents With ADHD

Table 3–1 provides an overview of studies examining the comorbidity of ADHD with mood, antisocial, and anxiety disorders.

Major Depression

ADHD and mood disorders have been found to co-occur in 15%–
75% of cases in both epidemiological and clinical samples of children and adolescents (Biederman et al. 1991c). Some investigators,

Table 3–1. Summary of representative studies of the comorbidity of attention-deficit/hyperactivity disorder (ADHD) with antisocial, mood, and anxiety disorders

Total no. of studies	No. by type of study	Year range	Subject age range (years)	Number of subjects	Findings
ADHD-positive antisocial disorders					
27	R = 18 N = 9	1979–1991	4–25	8,036	• In ADHD, overlap with antisocial disorders ranged from 23%–64% in referred and from 47%–57% in nonreferred children • In antisocial disorders, overlap with ADHD reported as 85% in one study of referred children and ranged from 35%–47% in nonreferred children • All but one study reported at least some differences between ADHD and antisocial disorders • ADHD-positive conduct disorder is a more severe subtype of ADHD
ADHD-positive mood disorders					
18	R = 16 N = 2	1973–1989	4–33	3,344	• In ADHD, overlap with mood disorders ranged from 25%–75% in referred and from 15%–19% in nonreferred children • In mood disorders, overlap with ADHD reported as 55% in one study of referred children and ranged from 30%–57% in nonreferred children • 78% of studies reported higher than expected rates of mood disorders in ADHD children

(continued)

Table 3–1. Summary of representative studies of the comorbidity of attention-deficit/hyperactivity disorder (ADHD) with antisocial, mood, and anxiety disorders *(continued)*

Total no. of studies	No. by type of study	Year range	Subject age range (years)	Number of subjects	Findings
ADHD-positive anxiety disorders					
11	R = 9 N = 2	1985–1991	4–23	2,259	• In ADHD, overlap with anxiety disorders ranged from 27%–30% in referred children and from 8%–26% in nonreferred samples
					• In anxiety disorders, overlap with ADHD reported as 18% in one study of referred children and ranged from 18%–24% in nonreferred children
					• All but two studies reported at least some overlap between ADHD and anxiety disorders

Note. ADHD = attention-deficit hyperactivity disorder; R = referred; N = nonreferred.
Source. Adapted from Biederman et al. 1991c.

however, have not found higher than expected rates of mood disorders in children with ADHD (Gittelman et al. 1985; Lahey et al. 1988a; Stewart and Morrison 1973; Weiss 1985). In clinical samples, the association between ADHD and mood disorders has been reported in studies of children with nonbipolar major depression and dysthymia (Alessi and Magen 1988), in adolescents with bipolar disorder (Strober et al. 1988), and in studies of children with ADHD (Biederman et al. 1990a; Bohline 1985; Brown et al. 1988; Munir et al. 1987). Studies of high-risk children of parents with mood disorders have found high rates of ADHD in these children (Keller et al. 1988; Orvaschel 1989; Orvaschel et al. 1988), and family studies of children with ADHD have found a significantly higher rate of mood disorders in children with ADHD and in their first-degree relatives compared with normal control children and their first-degree relatives (Biederman et al. 1987b). Studies of adopted children diagnosed with ADHD showed high rates of major depressive disorder in their biological relatives compared with their adoptive relatives and the biological relatives of control subjects (Deutsch et al. 1982). Recent case reports have described individuals with a childhood history of ADHD who developed major affective disorders in later years (Dvoredsky and Stewart 1981). It is doubtful that the comorbidity between ADHD and mood disorders can be explained by ascertainment bias, because high levels of comorbidity between ADHD and mood disorders have also been found in culturally and regionally diverse population-based epidemiological samples (Anderson et al. 1987; Bird et al. 1988; McGee et al. 1985).

Several investigators have presented data consistent with a familial link between ADHD and depression. Stewart and Morrison (1973) reported that rates of depression were similar between mothers of hyperactive probands and control subjects (9% vs. 10%), but there was a twofold greater rate of depression among the fathers of hyperactive probands versus fathers of control subjects (10% vs. 5%). Although this twofold difference was not significant, there was a statistically significant threefold increase in rates of depression among second-degree relatives of hyperactive probands compared with control subjects (6% vs. 2%). Welner et al. (1977) found significantly more depressive symptoms among the nonhyperactive brothers of hyperactive probands than among nonhyperactive control subjects. Rates of depression were not presented, but 36% of the brothers of hyperactive probands had three or more depressive symptoms compared with 6% of brothers of control subjects. This familial link with depression was not found for sisters. A similar pattern of results for parents was reported by Bhatia et al. (1991). Fathers of ADHD probands were at significantly greater risk for depression than were fathers of control subjects (7% vs. 2%), but rates in mothers were not significantly different (2% vs. 1%). Elevated rates of depression in parents of children with ADHD were also reported by R. Schachar (personal communication, May 1993) and by Schachar and Wachsmuth (1990). Levy and Nurcombe (1979) found that, compared with mothers of healthy control subjects, mothers of hyperactive children had significantly higher levels of depressed mood and anxiety. Barkley et al. (1991) reported that mothers of probands with both ADHD and oppositional defiant disorder had significantly higher levels of depression and phobic anxiety. However, mothers of ADHD probands without oppositional defiant disorder did not differ from mothers of normal control subjects.

The increased rates of depression seen in the families of children with ADHD suggest that the two disorders may share familial risk factors. This hypothesis also predicts increased rates of ADHD in the children of depressed parents. Such increased rates have been reported in some family studies (Orvaschel et al. 1988), but not others (Weissman et al. 1987). These conflicting results highlight the etiological complexities underlying psychiatric comorbidity and underscore the need for comorbidity assessments in studies of ADHD.

Findings reported by Biederman et al. (1991b) support the hypothesis that attention-deficit disorder (ADD) as defined in DSM-III (American Psychiatric Association 1980) and major depressive disorder may share common familial vulnerabilities. Familial risk analyses revealed the following:

■ The risk for major depressive disorder among the relatives of patients with ADD as defined in DSM-III was significantly higher than the risk to relatives of healthy comparison children.

▪ The risk for major depressive disorder was the same among the relatives of DSM-III–defined ADD children with and without major depressive disorder and was significantly higher in both groups than the risk to relatives of healthy control children
▪ The two disorders did not cosegregate within families.

These findings are consistent with the hypothesis that ADD as defined in DSM-III and major depressive disorder may represent a different expression of the same etiological factors responsible for the manifestation of DSM-III–defined ADD. The reasons why the shared genotype may have differing phenotypic expressions, such as DSM-III–defined ADD, major depressive disorder, or DSM-III–defined ADD with major depressive disorder, remains unknown.

Moreover, these findings were replicated in an independent sample of children with ADHD as defined in DSM-III-R (American Psychiatric Association 1987; Biederman et al. 1992). The risks for ADHD among relatives of children with ADHD who also had major depressive disorder and ADHD children without major depressive disorder did not differ significantly from one another (21% vs. 14%) but were higher than the risk to relatives of control subjects (3%). The risks for major depressive disorder among relatives of children with ADHD who also had major depressive disorder and ADHD children without major depressive disorder did not differ significantly from one another (20% vs. 15%) but were higher than the risk to relatives of control subjects (9%). These findings are consistent with the idea that ADHD and major depressive disorder share common familial risk factors.

Conduct Disorder

ADHD and conduct disorder have been found to co-occur in 30%–50% of cases in both epidemiological and clinical samples (Biederman et al. 1991c). Two positions can be identified concerning the relationship between ADHD and conduct disorder. One suggests that ADHD and conduct disorder are indistinguishable (complete overlap), and the other suggests that they are either partially or completely independent. The position that ADHD and conduct disorder are indistinguishable suggests that, given the measurement and diagnosis of either ADHD or conduct disorder, the identification of the other yields no additional information. Proponents of this position point to the similarities between children with ADHD and those with conduct disorder frequently reported in studies of correlates, outcome, and treatment responses (Barkley et al. 1989; Quay et al. 1987). Similarly, they point to intercorrelations between symptoms of ADHD and those of conduct disorder (aggressive, disruptive, and noncompliant behaviors), which are often reported in factor analytic studies of children with behavior disorders (Campbell and Werry 1986; Quay 1986). In addition, they cite a lack of significant differences in psychosocial, neurodevelopmental, and perinatal factors between children with ADHD and those with conduct disorder (Sandberg et al. 1980).

Support for the independent position can be derived from studies that compared patterns of familial aggregation, cognitive performance, and outcome between children with ADHD and those with ADHD plus conduct disorder. For example, in the studies of Loney et al. (1981), symptoms of hyperactivity and aggression were not highly correlated and showed different patterns of concurrent and predictive validity, suggesting that they were separate dimensions. In those studies, the presence of conduct disorder in childhood, whether associated with ADHD or not, was significantly correlated with aggressive behavior and delinquency in adolescence (Loney et al. 1981), whereas childhood ADHD without conduct disorder was correlated with cognitive and academic deficits (Milich and Loney 1979; Stewart et al. 1980; Szatmari et al. 1989). Similar findings emerged from a follow-up study in a nonclinical sample (McGee et al. 1984a, 1984b).

Based on a family study of children with ADHD, we proposed that children with ADHD plus conduct disorder might be a distinct genetic subtype of ADHD (Faraone et al. 1991b). This conclusion was based on the fact that, among relatives of children with ADHD, conduct and antisocial personality disorders were primarily seen in the families of children with ADHD plus conduct disorders. We replicated this work in an independent sample of children with ADHD as defined in DSM-III-R (Biederman et al. 1992). The risks for ADHD among relatives of children who had ADHD with conduct disorder and those who had ADHD without conduct disorder did not differ significantly from one another (19% vs. 15%) but were higher than the risk to relatives of control subjects (3%). The risks for conduct disorder or antisocial personality disorder among relatives of children with ADHD plus conduct disorder were two times higher than the risk to relatives of children who had ADHD without conduct disorder (26% vs. 13%). Both were higher than the risk to relatives of control subjects (8%); however, the difference was significant for ADHD plus conduct disorder and not significant for ADHD without conduct disorder. Among families of children with ADHD plus conduct disorder, we found that relatives of these children were significantly more likely to have one or more antisocial disorder if they also had the diagnosis of ADHD (39% vs. 10%). That is, ADHD and antisocial disorders cosegregated (i.e., were not independently transmitted) in the families of children with ADHD plus conduct disorder. These findings are most consistent with the idea that ADHD plus conduct disorder is familially distinct from ADHD without conduct disorder.

Thus, stratification by conduct disorder may cleave the universe of ADHD children into more genetically homogeneous subgroups. In contrast, major depression may be a nonspecific manifestation of different ADHD subforms. Data from other groups also favored a familial distinction between children who had ADHD with conduct disorder and other children with ADHD. Stewart et al. (1980) found alcoholic or antisocial disorders to be more frequent among fathers of unsocialized, aggressive, hyperactive boys compared with fathers of boys who were only hyperactive. Lahey et al. (1988b) reported higher rates of antisocial disorders, depression, and substance abuse among relatives of probands with ADHD plus conduct disorder compared with other ADHD probands. Their data indicated that the risk for depression in relatives of children with ADHD was most prominent when the child had conduct disorder. Similarly, Barkley et al. (1991) reported that mothers of probands with both ADHD and oppositional defiant disorder had significantly higher levels of depression and phobic anxiety. However, mothers of ADHD probands without oppositional defiant disorder did not differ from mothers of healthy control subjects.

In another study, the mothers of children with ADHD plus conduct disorder were found to have higher rates of psychopathology (as measured by the Minnesota Multiphasic Personality Inventory) than the mothers of other ADHD children (Lahey et al. 1989). In a study by Frick et al. (1991a), parents of children with ADHD plus conduct disorder had higher rates of childhood hyperactivity, conduct disorder, and substance use than parents of other ADHD children. August and Stewart (1983) reported that, among hyperactive children, a family history of hyperactivity predicted more symptoms of conduct disorder in the child and a greater risk of conduct disorder to siblings. Overall, these data suggest that, from a familial perspective, children with ADHD plus conduct disorder may be etiologically distinct from those without conduct disorder.

In contrast to the well-grounded nosological status of conduct disorder, that of oppositional defiant disorder—and, consequently, that of ADHD plus oppositional defiant disorder—remains unclear (Popper 1988; Werry et al. 1987). To date, only a few studies have generated data on oppositional defiant disorder. Some of these studies have grouped oppositional defiant disorder and conduct disorder together into a single antisocial behavioral category, making it difficult to draw conclusions about oppositional defiant disorder itself. The few studies available report an overlap of at least 35% between ADHD and oppositional defiant disorder, either alone or combined with conduct disorder, in both epidemiological studies (Anderson et al. 1987; Bird et al. 1988) and clinical studies (Biederman et al. 1990a; Faraone et al. 1991b) of children and adolescents. Faraone et al. (1991b) demonstrated that oppositional disorder itself, as defined in DSM-III, is also familial, with a risk for oppositional disorder among relatives of children with DSM-III–defined ADD plus oppositional disorder being three times greater than the risk to relatives of children with DSM-III–defined ADD without oppositional disorder and nearly 10 times greater than the risk to relatives of healthy control subjects. These data provide some evidence for the validity of DSM-III–defined oppositional disorder. In terms of severity of the clinical picture, the available data suggest that children with ADHD plus oppositional defiant disorder may form an intermediate subgroup between those who have ADHD alone and those who have ADHD plus conduct disorder. For example, Faraone et al. (1991b) showed that, whereas children who have ADD as defined in DSM-III plus oppositional disorder had a higher rate of school dysfunction than those with DSM-III–defined ADD alone, this rate was lower than that of the subgroup of individuals who had ADD as defined in DSM-III plus conduct disorder. These findings are consistent with the hypothesis that oppositional defiant disorder may be a subsyndromal manifestation of conduct disorder (Loney 1985).

Anxiety Disorders

A comorbid association of approximately 25% between ADHD and anxiety disorders has been found in epidemiological and clinical samples of children with anxiety disorders and children with ADHD (Biederman et al. 1991c). Investigators have also noted higher rates of ADHD in children of parents with anxiety disorders than in children of comparison groups (Sylvester et al. 1987). Lahey et al. (1987, 1988a) noted that children with the DSM-III diagnosis of ADD without hyperactivity had higher rates of anxiety disorders than those with ADHD. Our investigation (Biederman et al. 1991a) of the familial interrelationship between ADHD and anxiety disorders provides evidence for an association between the two disorders as follows. First, the risk for anxiety disorders among the relatives of patients with ADHD was significantly higher than the risk to relatives of healthy comparison children. Second, the risk for anxiety disorders was significantly higher in relatives of children with ADHD and anxiety disorders compared with relatives of children with ADHD without anxiety disorders. Finally, cosegregation between ADHD and anxiety disorders within families could not be established. These findings suggest that ADHD and anxiety disorders transmit independently in families.

We found similar results in our DSM-III-R sample (Biederman et al. 1992). The risks for ADHD among relatives of children with ADHD plus multiple anxiety disorders and ADHD children without them did not differ significantly from one another (18% vs. 16%), but were higher than the risk to relatives of control subjects (3%). The risk for multiple anxiety disorders among relatives of children with ADHD plus multiple anxiety disorders was 50% higher than the risk to relatives of children with ADHD without multiple anxi-

ety disorders (29% vs. 19%). Both were higher than the risk to relatives of control subjects (13%); however, the difference was highly
significant for children with ADHD plus multiple anxiety disorders
and only marginally significant for ADHD without multiple anxiety
disorders. ADHD and anxiety disorders did not cosegregate among
relatives of children with ADHD plus multiple anxiety disorders.
These results are most consistent with the hypothesis that ADHD
and anxiety disorders are independently transmitted.

Cognitive Performance and Learning Disabilities

Academic difficulties have often been found to co-occur with
ADHD (Biederman et al. 1991c). Inattentiveness, excessive motor
activity, impulsivity, and distractibility have been associated with
poor academic development (Cantwell 1985; Levine et al. 1982;
Silver and Brunstetter 1986; Weiss et al. 1979). Studies have consistently shown that children with ADHD perform more poorly in
school than do control subjects, as evidenced by more grade repe-
titions, poorer grades in academic subjects, more placement in special classes, and more tutoring (Edelbrock et al. 1984; Faraone et
al. 1993a, 1993b; Lahey et al. 1984; Semrud-Clikeman et al. 1992;
Silver 1981; Weiss et al. 1979). Findings also indicate that children
with ADHD perform more poorly than do control subjects on
standard measures of intelligence and achievement (Campbell and
Werry 1986).

Although children with ADHD may show learning disabilities,
these two disorders are not mutually inclusive (Gaddes 1983).
A widely variable overlap between ADHD and learning disabilities
has been reported in the literature (Biederman et al. 1991c; Semrud-Clikeman et al. 1992). The reported degree of overlap ranges
from as low as 10% (August and Holmes 1984; Halperin et al. 1984)
to as high as 92% (Silver 1981). This variability is most likely due
to differences in selection criteria, sampling, and measurement instruments, as well as inconsistencies in the criteria used to define
both ADHD and learning disabilities in different studies (August
and Garfinkel 1989; Halperin and Gittelman 1982).

A summary of the pertinent literature on ADHD and learning
disabilities (as reviewed by Semrud-Clikeman et al. 1992) is shown

in Table 3–2. These studies used inconsistent criteria for learning disabilities. Some of the cited studies do not report IQ (Holborow and Berry 1986; Levine et al. 1982; Silver 1981), which makes it difficult to ascertain whether their groups are equal in ability. The studies that do not report IQ also do not determine the presence of a disability in relation to the child's ability. Moreover, results from achievement tests are not reported in several studies (Levine et al. 1982; Silver 1981) or are combined to determine a learning disability (Holborow and Berry 1986). Out of 11 studies reviewed, only 6 utilized a comparison between ability and achievement (August and Holmes 1984; Barkley 1990; Frick et al. 1991b; Halperin et al. 1984; Lambert and Sandoval 1980; McGee et al. 1984b). A major point of the learning disabilities definition is a significant discrepancy between aptitude and achievement in one or more subject areas. The lack of utility of this major element of recognized learning disabilities criteria in 46% of the studies makes interpretation of results across studies difficult at best.

Several conclusions may be drawn from this overview of representative studies. The percentage of children with ADHD and concomitant learning disabilities may be inflated because of methodological problems in several of the studies. Most of the studies did not utilize careful diagnostic parameters for learning disabilities criteria. In fact, five studies did not utilize achievement data for determination of the presence of a learning disability (Levine et al. 1982; Nussbaum et al. 1990; Schachar et al. 1981; Silver 1981). In contrast, studies that attempted to control for intelligence variables as well as psychopathology found rates of learning disabilities between 7% and 43% among hyperactive children (August and Holmes 1984; Lambert and Sandoval 1980; McGee et al. 1984b), a far cry from the 66%–92% incidence rate quoted in other studies (Levine et al. 1982; Silver 1981). Frick et al. (1991b) compared three methods of determining the existence of academic underachievement in groups with ADHD, conduct disorder, and ADD without hyperactivity. The findings in this study were significantly lower than many of the other studies reviewed in Table 3–2.

Semrud-Clikeman et al. (1992) compared three methods for determining the presence of a learning disability in a sample of clinically referred children with DSM-III–defined ADHD. They found

Table 3–2. Summary of comorbidity of attention-deficit/hyperactivity disorder with learning disabilities

Year range	Diagnostic groups studied	Number of subjects	Rates of learning disabilities (%)
Epidemiologic and school samples			
1980–1986	Hyperactive/DSM-III attention-deficit disorder	575	3–43
	Conduct disorder/behavioral disorders	86	0–19
	Hyperactive + conduct disorder	46	27–37
	Control	3,650	2–11
Referred samples			
1981–1991	Hyperactive/DSM-III attention-deficit disorder/DSM-III-R attention-deficit hyperactivity disorder	1,369	6–92
	Conduct disorder/behavioral disorders	68	6–18
	Hyperactive/DSM-III attention-deficit disorder/DSM-III-R attention-deficit hyperactivity disorder + conduct disorder	58	8–47
	Emotional disturbance/pervasive developmental delay	333	4–59
	Control	130	0–35
Summary			
	Hyperactive/DSM-III attention-deficit disorder/DSM-III-R attention-deficit hyperactivity disorder	1,944	3–92
	Conduct disorder/behavioral disorders	154	0–19
	Hyperactive/DSM-III attention-deficit disorder/DSM-III-R attention-deficit hyperactivity disorder + conduct disorder	104	8–47
	Emotional disturbance/pervasive developmental delay	333	4–59
	Control	3,780	0–35

Source. Adapted from Semrud-Clikeman et al. 1992.

significant differences between children with ADHD, children with academic problems, and healthy control subjects using three different methods to assess reading disability. The first method (reading achievement score ≥10 standard score points below full-scale IQ), found reading disability among 38% of the ADHD sample, 43% of the children with academic problems, and 8% of healthy control subjects. Their second method (reading achievement score ≥20 standard score points below full-scale IQ) produced rates of 23% for the subjects with ADHD, 10% for the children with academic problems, and 2% for the healthy control subjects. The third method (reading achievement score ≤85 and ≥15 standard score points below full-scale IQ) found reading disability among 15% of the subjects with ADHD, 3% of the children with academic problems, and 0% of the healthy control subjects. Although the absolute rates of reading disability were sensitive to the method of definition, the differences between subjects with ADHD and control subjects remained significant for each definition.

Faraone et al. (1993a) examined ADHD and learning disabilities among the first-degree relatives of ADHD probands and control subjects. Their first finding was that the risks for ADHD among the relatives of ADHD probands with and without learning disabilities was significantly higher than the risk for ADHD among the relatives of healthy comparison probands. Their second finding was that the risk for learning disabilities was elevated only among relatives of probands with ADHD plus learning disabilities. Their third finding was that ADHD and learning disabilities did not cosegregate among the relatives of probands with ADHD plus learning disabilities. Their final finding was that there was nonrandom mating between ADHD and spouses with learning disability. These findings suggest that ADHD and learning disabilities are etiologically independent but co-occur due to nonrandom mating. The results were not compatible with the idea that ADHD and learning disabilities are manifestations of a single disorder or with the hypothesis that patients with ADHD plus learning disabilities are children with ADHD who develop learning disabilities secondary to the symptomatology of ADHD. These data are also not consistent with the hypothesis that ADHD plus learning disabilities is etiologically distinct from ADHD without learning disabilities.

Faraone et al.'s (1993a) finding of the independent transmission between ADHD and learning disabilities is consistent with a twin study of these conditions (Gilger et al. 1992). The cross concordances between ADHD and learning disabilities were 44% for monozygotic twins and 30% for dizygotic twins. The small difference between monozygotic and dizygotic twins led the authors to conclude that ADHD and learning disabilities were, for the most part, genetically independent.

The interpretation of cognitive and school difficulties among children with ADHD is complicated by the comorbidity of ADHD with other psychiatric disorders. For example, a large body of literature shows academic underachievement to be associated with dimensional assessments of externalizing behavior problems. These data are reviewed comprehensively by Hinshaw (1992). This association, seen in both epidemiological and clinical studies, exceeds the chance expectation. Furthermore, there appears to be a developmental progression: at younger ages, neuropsychological disability is primarily associated with hyperactivity and inattention; for older children, there is a stronger link with aggressiveness and antisocial behavior (Hinshaw 1992).

The internalizing disorders found comorbidly with ADHD are also linked to academic underachievement and neuropsychological dysfunction. Depressed children have lower intelligence test scores and poor performance in school (Frost et al. 1989; Hodges and Plow 1990). Self-report, peer, and teacher ratings of depression predict ratings of academic incompetence among schoolchildren unselected for psychopathology (Cole 1990). Anxious children do poorly on tasks requiring complex problem solving and visual motor integration (Frost et al. 1989). They also achieve lower scores on global measures of intelligence (Hodges and Plow 1990).

Several studies clarify the impact of psychiatric comorbidity on neuropsychological dysfunction. Frost et al. (1989) examined neuropsychological functioning in an unselected cohort of young adolescents. They found evidence of neuropsychological impairment among children with ADHD. However, in the absence of comorbid ADHD, children with conduct disorder or depression were similar to healthy control subjects. Similar results emerged from Frick et al.'s (1991b) study of academic underachievement in children with ADHD and conduct disorder. They found an association between school failure and conduct disorder, but this could be accounted for by the comorbidity of conduct disorder with ADHD. Thus, some intellectual impairments appear to be core features of the ADHD syndrome, not epiphenomena of disruptive behavior or other psychiatric syndromes.

Faraone et al. (1993b) found that the neuropsychological impairments of their ADHD sample were due to the ADHD syndrome itself; they could not be accounted for by psychiatric comorbidity. Among subjects with ADHD, comorbid conduct disorders and major depressive and anxiety disorders predicted placement in special classes but tutoring, repeated grades, or learning disabilities did not predict such placement. Psychiatric comorbidity also had limited influence on Wechsler Intelligence Scale for Children—Revised (WISC-R) scores. Among ADHD probands, psychiatric comorbidity was significantly associated with block design scores and full-scale IQ. ADHD with depression predicted higher scores than ADHD-only on both block design measures and full-scale IQ measures, whereas conduct and anxiety disorders predicted lower scores.

▼ Comorbidity in Adult ADHD

Although ADHD was originally conceptualized as a childhood disorder, it is also seen in adults. Follow-up studies find that 30%–50% of children with ADHD continue to have ADHD as adults (Gittelman et al. 1985; Weiss 1985), and family genetic studies show that many parents and adult siblings of children with ADHD also have ADHD (Biederman et al. 1990a, 1992; Faraone et al. 1991a). Moreover, like children with ADHD, many clinically referred adults with ADHD benefit from stimulant therapy (Spencer et al. 1992; Wender et al. 1981). However, adult ADHD is not recognized in the official nomenclature and is an infrequent topic of investigation. Nevertheless, there are some data that speak to the issue of psychiatric comorbidity. Two sources are available: cross-sectional studies of adults diagnosed with ADHD and follow-up studies into adulthood of children with ADHD.

Cross-Sectional Studies of Adults

Psychiatric Disorders

The early studies of ADHD, which employed nonblind, clinical assessments for diagnoses, consistently found comorbidity in their samples. Borland and Heckman (1976) reported high rates of antisocial personality, anxiety, and depressive disorders among adults with childhood-only ADHD as well as those with childhood-onset adult ADHD. Morrison (1980a, 1980b) compared outpatient adults having childhood-onset ADHD ($N = 48$) to psychiatric control subjects. Although they did not assess for the persistence of ADHD, the authors reported that the ADHD group had higher rates of antisocial personality disorder and alcoholism as adults.

Several early studies of adults with substance abuse disorders found significantly elevated rates of childhood ADHD (Alterman et al. 1982; DeObaldia and Pasons 1984; Eyre et al. 1982; Goodwin et al. 1975; Tarter 1982) as well as childhood-onset adult ADHD (Cocores et al. 1987; Gomez et al. 1981; Wood et al. 1983) compared with control subjects. For example, Goodwin et al. (1975) reported a 50% rate of childhood ADHD in adopted adults with alcoholism and only 15% among adopted adults who did not have alcoholism. The alcoholic adults with ADHD also had higher rates of poor school performance. Other investigators (Alterman et al. 1982; DeObaldia and Pasons 1984; Eyre et al. 1982; Tarter 1982) found that compared with adults who only have substance use disorders, adults with substance use disorders who also had a history of childhood ADHD showed characteristics frequently encountered among children and adolescents with ADHD: social maladjustment, immaturity, personality disturbance, lower social assets, less ego capacity to regulate drives, impulse control deficits, and school failure. These ADHD-type problems persisted into adulthood and were associated with poor academic and occupational achievement, high rates of separation and divorce, and social impairment.

Treatment studies of adults with ADHD also report psychiatric comorbidity (Gualtieri et al. 1985; Mattes et al. 1984; Spencer et al. 1992; Wender et al. 1981, 1985; Wilens and Biederman 1992; Wood et al. 1976). The adults with ADHD in these studies had high rates of substance abuse (27%–46%), antisocial personality disorders (12%–27%), and anxiety disorders (50%). More recently, Biederman et al. (1993) reported that adults with ADHD had high rates of antisocial, mood, and anxiety disorders.

Biederman et al. (1993) studied 84 referred adults of both sexes. Each had a clinical diagnosis of childhood-onset ADHD confirmed by structured interview. They also studied the 43 nonreferred adult relatives of ADHD children from a preexisting sample (Biederman et al. 1992). Compared with control subjects, the referred and nonreferred adults with ADHD had significantly higher rates of antisocial, substance use, and anxiety disorders, enuresis, stuttering, and speech and language disorders.

The high levels of psychiatric comorbidity in adults with ADHD are consistent with findings reported in children and adolescents with ADHD. Although this consistent pattern of comorbidity strengthens evidence for descriptive validity, skeptics may raise the question of whether the adult form is merely secondary to these (or other) psychiatric disorders. If so, it may be that childhood ADHD is a neurodevelopmental precursor to other disorders: the childhood symptoms of inattention, impulsivity, and hyperactivity do not represent a distinct disorder with a predictable course but are only a prodrome to a more typical disorder, such as depression, whose characteristic features may not fully emerge until adulthood. This issue has not been systematically addressed in previous studies of adult ADHD and remains a priority for research. However, some data do speak to this issue.

If adult ADHD is secondary to other disorders it should rarely be present without a comorbid psychiatric disorder. This was not the case in the studies reviewed above. In these studies, approximately 40% of adults with ADHD did not have a comorbid psychiatric disorder. For example, in the study by Biederman et al. (1993), 23% of the adults with ADHD had no adult psychiatric disorder, yet met full DSM-III-R criteria for ADHD in childhood and had the characteristic symptoms of inattentiveness, distractibility, and impulsivity associated with ADHD. Compared with normal control adults, the condition of uncomplicated ADHD was also associated with significant impairment, consistent with the status of being a meaningful psychiatric disorder. These impairments were evidenced by poorer functioning on the Global Assessment of Functioning scale, and poorer cognitive performance, as evidenced by history of school failure and impaired performance on neuropsychological measures (Biederman et al. 1993).

Cognitive Performance and Learning Disabilities

Given that the cognitive correlates of ADHD in children are pervasive and disabling, one would expect to find similar findings in adults who apparently have the same disorder. Results from standardized, individually administered psychological tests would be particularly useful because such data are less likely than interview data to be contaminated by reporter biases. Unfortunately, there is very little systematically collected data about the intellectual performance of adults with ADHD. Two studies by Biederman et al. (1990b, 1993) examined school failure (repeated grades, need for academic tutoring, and placement in special classes) and performance on subtests of the Wechsler Adult Intelligence Scale—Revised (WAIS-R) (Wechsler 1981). Because children and adolescents with ADHD are at high risk for alcohol and substance abuse, more work needs to be done to determine the potential contribution of substance abuse disorders to cognitive performance. However, whereas these studies did not specifically investigate this issue, adults with ADHD showed more evidence of school failure and had lower cognitive test scores than adults without ADHD.

Follow-Up Studies of Children With ADHD

The most sophisticated follow-up studies used operationalized, DSM-III–based criteria, comparison groups, and blind assessments to examine adults who had childhood-onset ADHD (Gittelman et al. 1985; Greenfield et al. 1988; Mannuzza et al. 1991; Weiss 1985). These studies clearly documented the reliability of the diagnosis of ADHD in adults. These adults had symptoms of inattention, disorganization, distractibility, and impulsiveness. These symptoms were associated with significant difficulties not only in childhood but also in adulthood (i.e., significant social and occupational impairment).

Although the study designs, methods of ascertainment, and diagnostic criteria vary among longitudinal studies of children with

ADHD, most report high rates (30%–60%) of ADHD symptoms in adolescence (Klein and Mannuzza 1989, 1991; Thorley 1984; Weiss and Hechtman 1986) and adulthood (Gittelman et al. 1985; Greenfield et al. 1988; Mannuzza et al. 1991; Weiss et al. 1985). For example, Weiss et al. (1985), Greenfield et al. (1988), Gittelman et al. (1985), and Mannuzza et al. (1991) found that 31%–44% of young adults with childhood-onset ADHD had the full syndrome, and 9%–25% had a partial syndrome with at least one disabling symptom. These high rates of persistent ADHD were clinically and statistically higher than the 3%–10% (Gittelman et al. 1985; Mannuzza et al. 1991; Weiss 1985) found in healthy control subjects. In a later follow-up of their sample, Gittelman et al. (1985) and Mannuzza et al. (1993) reported a rate of persistence of ADHD symptoms in adulthood (mean age 26 years) greater than that of control subjects (11% vs. 1%).

Follow-up data also indicate that many of the childhood correlates of ADHD persist with the disorder into adulthood. These include psychosocial dysfunction, school-related problems, work failure, and psychiatric comorbidity (especially substance abuse and antisocial personality) (Klein and Mannuzza 1989, 1991; Thorley 1984; Weiss and Hechtman 1986). For example, Weiss et al. (1979) and Klein and Mannuzza (1989) independently reported that adults with childhood ADHD were less educated, had poorer marks, failed more grades, and were more commonly expelled from school than control subjects. Klein and Mannuzza (1989) also reported that adults with ADHD had worse scores on standardized achievement tests (after controlling for intelligence).

Weiss et al. (1979) reported that adults with childhood ADHD had significant occupational impairment in adulthood. The employers of these adults said they had poor levels of work performance, impairment in task completion, lack of independent skills, and poor relationships with supervisors. This level of school and occupational problems seen in adults with ADHD is consistent with a vast literature indicating school and functional deficits in children and adolescents with the disorder (Barkley et al. 1990; Biederman et al. 1990a; Campbell and Werry 1986; Cantwell 1985; Edelbrock et al. 1984; Lahey et al. 1984; Levine et al. 1982; Silver 1981; Weiss et al. 1979).

The follow-up studies suggest that children with ADHD with an associated childhood onset of conduct disorder have a more serious clinical course and poorer outcome into adulthood than do children who have ADHD without conduct disorder (August and Holmes 1984; August et al. 1983; Farrington et al. 1989; Milich et al. 1987; Reeves et al. 1987; Robins 1966; Szatmari et al. 1989). Because follow-up studies of children and adolescents diagnosed with conduct disorder are in agreement regarding the strong predictive power of conduct disorder for future psychiatric disorders, social adjustment problems, antisocial personality, alcoholism, and criminality (Robins 1966), it has been suggested that the delinquent behaviors and substance abuse often reported in follow-up studies of boys with ADHD (Gittelman et al. 1985; Weiss 1985) may be linked to childhood antisocial disorders rather than to the syndrome of ADHD per se (August and Stewart 1983; Farrington et al. 1989; Mannuzza et al. 1989).

In contrast to the findings for conduct disorder, longitudinal studies have not reported children with ADHD to be at risk for mood and anxiety disorders, nor have they shown that anxiety or depression are robust predictors of adult outcome. However, it would seem premature to attribute all of the poor outcome of children with ADHD to conduct disorder alone. Many of the follow-up studies of children with ADHD started before current knowledge about the extensive comorbidity of ADHD with other disorders. As a result, their assessment of anxiety and depression may not have been comprehensive, especially as addressed from the perspective of lifetime history.

Moreover, follow-up data of children with ADHD as well as those with major depressive disorder (Kovacs et al. 1984, 1988) strongly suggest that, whereas these disorders are individually associated with significant long-term psychiatric morbidity, their co-occurrence may be associated with a particularly poor outcome. In a study that evaluated predictors of suicide in adolescents, Brent et al. (1988) reported that adolescents who committed suicide had increased rates of bipolarity and ADHD in comparison with those who attempted suicide. Thus, the co-occurrence of ADHD and a mood disorder is suggestive of a subpopulation of ADHD children at higher risk for greater psychiatric morbidity and disability (Weinberg et al. 1989), and perhaps at higher risk for suicide than are other children and adolescents with ADHD who lack such comorbidity.

▼ Implications of Comorbidity

Comorbidity complicates studies of ADHD. When two disorders co-occur, the correlates and outcomes of one disorder might be erroneously attributed to the other (Caron and Rutter 1991). For example, the three disorders most frequently associated with ADHD—conduct, depressive, and anxiety disorders—are also associated with intellectual disability. For example, children with conduct disorder often have deficits in verbal skills (Hodges et al. 1982, 1990; Ollendick 1979) and, less consistently, impairments in visuospatial, motor, memory, and executive functions (Frost et al. 1989; Hinshaw 1992; Moffitt and Silva 1988). Careful studies of children with and without comorbidity are needed to disentangle the causes and correlates of each disorder.

Moreover, subgroups of patients with ADHD and comorbid disorders may represent more homogeneous subgroups within ADHD. The strongest example of this is the subgroup of children with both ADHD and conduct disorder. We now know that these children are at high risk for additional comorbid disorders, familial psychopathology, and criminality. Subgrouping of children with ADHD along these lines, or others, may clarify research results. In particular, such subgrouping may be needed to permit the development of early intervention strategies for specific subgroups.

Comorbidity also has implications for clinical practice as a result of its influence on diagnosis, prognosis, treatment, and health care delivery (Maser and Cloninger 1990). The implications for diagnostic practice are clear: clinicians should not approach the diagnosis of children in a hierarchical fashion. The presence of one disorder does not automatically exclude others. In fact, it increases the likelihood that another is present. Given the extensive comorbidity of ADHD with major depression, conduct, and anxiety disorders, ADHD children should be routinely examined for the presence of comorbid conditions.

Thus, in diagnosing children with ADHD, one must be careful

not to dismiss other symptomatology as secondary. For example, it is not difficult to come up with reasons why an adolescent with ADHD might be depressed. Poor social skills, problems with parents, low academic functioning, and other correlates of ADHD can be construed as causal factors. Although these should not be ignored, neither should the possibility that the child has a major depressive disorder that might be responsive to appropriate pharmacotherapy.

A final diagnostic maxim that comes from studies of comorbidity is that the family, not the child, should be the unit of diagnostic analysis. A careful family history of most children with ADHD will uncover anxiety, depression, and antisocial disorders among immediate relatives. Although the predictive significance of these disorders among relatives is not yet known, it is reasonable to assume that if the disorder appears in the family, the child is at increased risk for its expression.

▼ References

American Psychiatric Association: Diagnostic and Statistic Manual of Mental Disorders, 3rd Edition. Washington, DC, American Psychiatric Association, 1980

American Psychiatric Association: Diagnostic and Statistic Manual of Mental Disorders, 3rd Edition, Revised. Washington, DC, American Psychiatric Association, 1987

Achenbach TM: Taxonomy and comorbidity of conduct problems: evidence from empirically based approaches. Development and Psychopathology 5:51–64, 1993

Alessi N, Magen J: Comorbidity of other psychiatric disturbances in depressed, psychiatrically hospitalized children. Am J Psychiatry 145:1582–1584, 1988

Alterman AI, Petrarulo E, Tarter R, et al: Hyperactivity and alcoholism: familial and behavioral correlates. Addict Behav 7:413–421, 1982

Anderson JC, Williams S, McGee R, et al: DSM-III disorders in preadolescent children: prevalence in a large sample from the general population. Arch Gen Psychiatry 44:69–76, 1987

Angold A, Costello EJ: Depressive comorbidity in children and adolescents: empirical, theoretical and methodological issues. Am J Psychiatry 150:1779–1791, 1993

August GJ, Garfinkel BD: Behavioral and cognitive subtypes of ADHD. J Am Acad Child Adolesc Psychiatry 28:739–748, 1989

August GJ, Holmes CS: Behavior and academic achievement in hyperactive subgroups and learning-disabled boys. Am J Dis Child 138:1025–1029, 1984

August GJ, Stewart MA: Familial subtypes of childhood hyperactivity. J Nerv Ment Dis 171:362–368, 1983

August GJ, Stewart MA, Holmes CS: A four-year follow-up of hyperactive boys with and without conduct disorder. Br J Psychiatry 143:192–198, 1983

Barkley RA: Attention Deficit Hyperactivity Disorder: A Handbook for Diagnosis and Treatment. New York, Guilford, 1990

Barkley RA, McMurray MB, Edelbrock CS, et al: The response of aggressive and nonaggressive ADHD children to two doses of methylphenidate. J Am Acad Child Adolesc Psychiatry 28:873–881, 1989

Barkley RA, DuPaul GJ, McMurray MB: Comprehensive evaluation of attention deficit disorder with and without hyperactivity as defined by research criteria. J Consult Clin Psychol 58:775–798, 1990

Barkley RA, Fischer M, Edelbrock CS, et al: The adolescent outcome of hyperactive children diagnosed by research criteria, III: mother-child interactions, family conflicts and maternal psychopathology. J Child Psychol Psychiatry 32:233–255, 1991

Bhatia M, Nigam V, Bohra N, et al: Attention deficit disorder with hyperactivity among pediatric outpatients. J Child Psychol Psychiatry 32:297–306, 1991

Biederman J, Munir K, Knee D: Conduct and oppositional disorder in clinically referred children with attention deficit disorder: a controlled family study. J Am Acad Child Adolesc Psychiatry 26:724–727, 1987a

Biederman J, Munir K, Knee D, et al: High rate of affective disorders in probands with attention deficit disorder and in their relatives: a controlled family study. Am J Psychiatry 144:330–333, 1987b

Biederman J, Faraone SV, Keenan K, et al: Family genetic and psychosocial risk factors in DSM-III attention deficit disorder. J Am Acad Child Adolesc Psychiatry 29:526–533, 1990a

Biederman J, Faraone SV, Knee D, et al: Retrospective assessment of DSM-III attention deficit disorder in non-referred individuals. J Clin Psychiatry 51:102–107, 1990b

Biederman J, Faraone SV, Keenan K, et al: Familial association between attention deficit disorder (ADD) and anxiety disorder. Am J Psychiatry 148:251–256, 1991a

Biederman J, Faraone SV, Keenan K, et al: Evidence of familial association between attention deficit disorder and major affective disorders. Arch Gen Psychiatry 48:633–642, 1991b

Biederman J, Newcorn J, Sprich S: Comorbidity of attention deficit hyperactivity disorder with conduct, depressive, anxiety, and other disorders. Am J Psychiatry 148:564–577, 1991c

Biederman J, Faraone SV, Keenan K, et al: Further evidence for family genetic risk factors in attention deficit hyperactivity disorder (ADHD): patterns of comorbidity in probands and relatives in psychiatrically and pediatrically referred samples. Arch Gen Psychiatry 49:728–738, 1992

Biederman J, Faraone SV, Spencer T, et al: Patterns of psychiatric comorbidity, cognition and psychosocial functioning in adults with attention deficit hyperactivity disorder. Am J Psychiatry 150:1792–1798, 1993

Bird HR, Canino G, Rubio-Stipec M, et al: Estimates of the prevalence of childhood maladjustment in a community survey in Puerto Rico. Arch Gen Psychiatry 45:1120–1126, 1988

Bohline DS: Intellectual and affective characteristics of attention deficit disordered children. Journal of Learning Disabilities 18:604–608, 1985

Borland BL, Heckman HK: Hyperactive boys and their brothers: a 25-year follow-up study. Arch Gen Psychiatry 33:669–675, 1976

Brent DA, Perper JA, Goldstein CE, et al: Risk factors for adolescent suicide: a comparison of adolescent suicide victims with suicidal inpatients. Arch Gen Psychiatry 45:581–588, 1988

Brown RT, Borden KA, Clingerman SR, et al: Depression in attention deficit-disordered and normal children and their parents. Child Psychiatry Hum Dev 18:119–132, 1988

Campbell SB, Werry JS: Attention deficit disorder (hyperactivity), in Psychopathologic Disorders of Childhood. Edited by Quay HC, Werry JS. New York, Wiley, 1986, pp 1–35

Cantwell DP: Hyperactive children have grown up: what have we learned about what happens to them? Arch Gen Psychiatry 42:1026–1028, 1985

Caron C, Rutter M: Comorbidity in child psychopathology: concepts, issues and research strategies. J Child Psychol Psychiatry 32:1063–1080, 1991

Cocores JA, Davies RK, Mueller PS, et al: Cocaine abuse and adult attention deficit disorder. J Clin Psychiatry 48:376–377, 1987

Cole DA: Relation of social and academic competence to depressive symptoms in childhood. J Abnorm Psychol 99:422–429, 1990

DeObaldia R, Pasons OA: Relationship of neuropsychological performance to primary alcoholism and self-reported symptoms of childhood minimal brain dysfunction. J Stud Alcohol 45:386–391, 1984

Deutsch CK, Swanson JM, Bruell JH, et al: Overrepresentation of adoptees in children with the attention deficit disorder. Behav Genet 12:231–238, 1982

Dvoredsky A, Stewart M: Hyperactivity followed by manic depressive disorder: two case reports. J Clin Psychiatry 42:212–214, 1981

Edelbrock C, Costello AJ, Kessler MD: Empirical corroboration of attention deficit disorder. J Am Acad Child Adolesc Psychiatry 23:285–290, 1984

Eyre S, Rounsaville B, Kleber H: History of childhood hyperactivity in a clinical population of opiate addicts. J Nerv Ment Dis 170:522–529, 1982

Faraone SV, Biederman J, Keenan K, et al: A family genetic study of girls with DSM-III attention deficit disorder. Am J Psychiatry 148:112–117, 1991a

Faraone SV, Biederman J, Keenan K, et al: Separation of DSM-III attention deficit disorder and conduct disorder: evidence from a family genetic study of American child psychiatric patients. Psychol Med 21:109–121, 1991b

Faraone S, Biederman J, Krifcher-Lehman B, et al: Evidence for the independent familial transmission of attention deficit hyperactivity disorder and learning disabilities: results from a family genetic study. Am J Psychiatry 150:891–895, 1993a

Faraone SV, Biederman J, Krifcher-Lehman B, et al: Intellectual performance and school failure in children with attention deficit hyperactivity disorder and in their siblings. J Abnorm Psychol 102:616–623, 1993b

Farrington DP, Loeber R, Van Kammen WB: Long-term criminal outcomes of hyperactivity-impulsivity-attention deficit and conduct problems in childhood, in Straight and Devious Pathways to Adulthood. Edited by Robbins LN, Rutter MR. New York, Cambridge University Press, 1989, pp 62–81

Frick PJ, Lahey BB, Christ MG, et al: History of childhood behavior problems in biological relatives of boys with attention deficit hyperactivity disorder and conduct disorder. Journal of Clinical Child Psychology 20:445–451, 1991a

Frick PJ, Lahey BB, Kamphaus RW, et al: Academic underachievement and the disruptive behavior disorders. J Consult Clin Psychol 59:289–294, 1991b

Frost LA, Moffitt TE, McGee R: Neuropsychological correlates of psychopathology in an unselected cohort of young adolescents. J Abnorm Psychol 98:307–313, 1989

Gaddes WH: Learning Disabilities and Brain Function: A Neuropsychological Approach. New York, Springer-Verlag New York, 1983

Gilger JW, Pennington BF, DeFries C: A twin study of the etiology of comorbidity: attention deficit hyperactivity disorder and dyslexia. J Am Acad Child Adolesc Psychiatry 31:343–348, 1992

Gittelman R, Mannuzza S, Shenker R, et al: Hyperactive boys almost grown up, I: psychiatric status. Arch Gen Psychiatry 42:937–947, 1985

Gomez RL, Janowsky D, Zetin M, et al: Adult psychiatric diagnosis and symptoms compatible with the hyperactive child syndrome: a retrospective study. J Clin Psychiatry 42:389–394, 1981

Goodwin D, Schulsinger F, Hermansen L, et al: Alcoholism and the hyperactive child syndrome. J Nerv Ment Dis 160:349–353, 1975

Greenfield B, Hechtman L, Weiss G: Two subgroups of hyperactives as adults: correlations of outcome. Can J Psychiatry 33:505–508, 1988

Gualtieri CT, Ondrusek MG, Finley C: Attention deficit disorders in adults. Clin Neuropharmacol 8:343–356, 1985

Halperin JM, Gittelman R: Do hyperactive children and their siblings differ in IQ and academic achievement? Psychiatry Res 6:253–258, 1982

Halperin JM, Gittelman R, Klein DF, et al: Reading-disabled hyperactive children: a distinct subgroup of attention deficit disorder with hyperactivity. J Abnorm Child Psychol 12:1–14, 1984

Hinshaw SP: Externalizing behavior problems and academic underachievement in childhood and adolescence: causal relationships and underlying mechanisms. Psychol Bull 111:127–155, 1992

Hodges K, Plow J: Intellectual ability and achievement in psychiatrically hospitalized children with conduct, anxiety, and affective disorders. J Consult Clin Psychol 58:589–595, 1990

Hodges K, Horowitz E, Kline J, et al: Comparison of various WISC-R summary scores for a psychiatric sample. J Clin Psychol 38:830–837, 1982

Hodges K, Saunders WB, Kashani J, et al: Internal consistency of DSM-III diagnoses using the symptom scales of the child assessment schedule. J Am Acad Child Adolesc Psychiatry 29:635–641, 1990

Holborow PL, Berry PS: Hyperactivity and learning difficulties. Journal of Learning Disabilities 19:426–431, 1986

Keller MB, Beardslee W, Lavori PW, et al: Course of major depression in non-referred adolescents: a retrospective study. J Affect Disord 15:235–243, 1988

Klein RG, Mannuzza S: The long-term outcome of the attention deficit disorder/hyperkinetic syndrome, in Attention Deficit Disorder, Clinical and Basic Research. Edited by Sagvolden T, Archer T. Hillside, NJ, Lawrence Erlbaum Associates, Inc, 1989, pp 71–91

Klein RG, Mannuzza S: Long-term outcome of hyperactive children: a review. J Am Acad Child Adolesc Psychiatry 30:383–387, 1991

Kovacs M, Feinberg TL, Crouse-Novak M, et al: Depressive disorders in childhood, I: a longitudinal prospective study of characteristics and recovery. Arch Gen Psychiatry 41:229–237, 1984

Kovacs M, Paulauskas S, Gatsonis C, et al: Depressive disorders in childhood, III: a longitudinal study of comorbidity with and risk for conduct disorders. J Affect Disord 15:205–217, 1988

Lahey BB, Schaughency EA, Strauss CC, et al: Are attention deficit disorders with and without hyperactivity similar or dissimilar disorders? J Am Acad Child Adolesc Psychiatry 23:302–309, 1984

Lahey BB, Schaughency EA, Hynd GW, et al: Attention deficit disorder with and without hyperactivity: comparison of behavioral characteristics of clinic-referred children. J Am Acad Child Adolesc Psychiatry 26:718–723, 1987

Lahey BB, Pelham WE, Schaughency EA, et al: Dimensions and types of attention deficit disorder. J Am Acad Child Adolesc Psychiatry 27:330–335, 1988a

Lahey BB, Piacentini JC, McBurnett K, et al: Psychopathology in the parents of children with conduct disorder and hyperactivity. J Am Acad Child Adolesc Psychiatry 27:163–170, 1988b

Lahey BB, Russo MF, Walker JL: Personality characteristics of the mothers of children with disruptive behavior disorders. J Consult Clin Psychol 57:512–515, 1989

Lambert NM, Sandoval J: The prevalence of learning disabilities in a sample of children considered hyperactive. J Abnorm Child Psychol 8:33–50, 1980

Leckman JF, Weissman MM, Merikangas KR, et al: Panic disorder and major depression: increased risk of depression, alcoholism, panic, and phobic disorders in families of depressed probands with panic disorder. Arch Gen Psychiatry 40:1055–1060, 1983

Levine MD, Busch B, Aufseeser C: The dimension of inattention among children with school problems. Pediatrics 70:387–395, 1982

Levy F, Nurcombe B: Depression and anxiety in the mothers of hyperactive children, in Genetic Aspects of Affective Illness: Current Concepts. Edited by Mendlewicz J, Shopsin B. New York, Luce Publications, 1979, pp 69–74

Loney J: Oppositional disorder: yes or no? Paper presented at the annual meeting of the American Academy of Child Psychiatry, San Antonio, TX, October 1985

Loney J, Kramer J, Milich RS: The hyperactive child grows up: predictors of symptoms, delinquency and achievement at follow-up, in Psychosocial Aspects of Drug Treatment for Hyperactivity. Edited by Gadow KD, Loney J. Boulder, CO, Westview Press, 1981, 381–416

Mannuzza S, Gittelman-Klein R, Horowitz-Konig P, et al: Hyperactive boys almost grown up, IV: criminality and its relationship to psychiatric status. Arch Gen Psychiatry 46:1073–1079, 1989

Mannuzza S, Gittelman Klein R, Bonagura N, et al: Hyperactive boys almost grown up, V: replication of psychiatric status. Arch Gen Psychiatry 48:77–83, 1991

Mannuzza S, Klein RG, Bessler A, et al: Adult outcome of hyperactive boys: educational achievement, occupational rank and psychiatric status. Arch Gen Psychiatry 50:565–576, 1993

Maser JD, Cloninger CR: Comorbidity of anxiety and mood disorders: introduction and overview, in Comorbidity of Mood and Anxiety Disorders. Edited by Maser JD, Cloninger CR. Washington, DC, American Psychiatric Press, 1990, pp 1–12

Mattes JA, Boswell L, Oliver H: Methylphenidate effects on symptoms of attention deficit disorder in adults. Arch Gen Psychiatry 41:1059–1063, 1984

McGee R, Williams S, Silva P: Background characteristics of aggressive, hyperactive and aggressive-hyperactive boys. J Am Acad Child Psychiatry 23:280–284, 1984a

McGee R, Williams S, Silva P: Behavioral and developmental characteristics of aggressive, hyperactive and aggressive-hyperactive boys. J Am Acad Child Psychiatry 23:270–279, 1984b

McGee R, Williams S, Silva P: Factor structure and correlates of ratings of inattention, hyperactivity, and antisocial behavior in a large sample of 9-year-old children from the general population. J Consult Clin Psychol 53:480–490, 1985

Milich R, Loney J: The role of hyperactive and aggressive symptomatology in predicting adolescent outcome among hyperactive children. J Pediatr Psychol 4:93–112, 1979

Milich R, Widiger TA, Landau S: Differential diagnosis of attention deficit and conduct disorders using conditional probabilities. J Consult Clin Psychol 55:762–767, 1987

Moffitt TE, Silva PA: Neuropsychological deficit and self-reported delinquency in an unselected birth cohort. J Am Acad Child Adolesc Psychiatry 27:233–240, 1988

Morrison JR: Adult psychiatric disorders in parents of hyperactive children. Am J Psychiatry 137:825–827, 1980a

Morrison JR: Childhood hyperactivity in an adult psychiatric population: social factors. J Clin Psychiatry 41:40–43, 1980b

Munir K, Biederman J, Knee D: Psychiatric comorbidity in patients with attention deficit disorder: a controlled study. J Am Acad Child Adolesc Psychiatry 26:844–848, 1987

Nussbaum NL, Grant ML, Roman MJ, et al: Attention deficit disorder and the mediating effect of age on academic and behavioral variables. Developmental and Behavioral Pediatrics 11:22–26, 1990

Ollendick TH: Discrepancies between verbal and performance IQs and subtest scatter on the WISC-R for juvenile delinquents. Psychol Rep 45:563–568, 1979

Orvaschel H: Comorbidity of attention deficit disorder and depression. Paper presented at the regional meeting of the World Federation of Societies of Biological Psychiatry, Jerusalem, Israel, April 1989

Orvaschel H, Walsh-Allis G, Ye W: Psychopathology in children of parents with recurrent depression. J Abnorm Child Psychol 16:17–28, 1988

Pauls DL, Hurst CR, Kruger SD, et al: Gilles de la Tourette's syndrome and attention deficit disorder with hyperactivity: evidence against a genetic relationship. Arch Gen Psychiatry 43:1177–1179, 1986a

Pauls DL, Towbin KE, Leckman JF, et al: Gilles de la Tourette's syndrome and obsessive-compulsive disorder: evidence supporting a genetic relationship. Arch Gen Psychiatry 43:1180–1182, 1986b

Popper CW: Disorders usually first evident in infancy, childhood or adolescence, in Textbook of Psychiatry. Edited by Talbott JA, Hales RE, Yudofsky SC. Washington, DC, American Psychiatric Press, 1988, pp 649–737

Quay HC: Conduct disorder, in Psychopathologic Disorders of Childhood. Edited by Quay HC, Werry JS. New York, Wiley, 1986, pp 35–73

Quay HC, Routh DK, Shapiro SK: Psychopathology of childhood: from description to validation. Annu Rev Psychol 38:491–532, 1987

Reeves JC, Werry JS, Elkind GS, et al: Attention deficit, conduct, oppositional, and anxiety disorders in children, II: clinical characteristics. J Am Acad Child Adolesc Psychiatry 26:144–155, 1987

Reich T, James J, Morris CA: The use of multiple thresholds in determining the mode of transmission of semi-continuous traits. Annals of Human Genetics 36:163–183, 1972

Reich T, Rice J, Cloninger CR, et al: The use of multiple thresholds and segregation analysis in analyzing the phenotypic heterogeneity of multifactorial traits. Annals of Human Genetics 42:371–389, 1979

Robins L: Deviant Children Grown Up. Baltimore, MD, Williams & Wilkins, 1966

Sandberg ST, Wieselberg M, Schaffer D: Hyperkinetic and conduct problem children in a primary school population: some epidemiological considerations. J Child Psychol Psychiatry 21:293–311, 1980

Schachar R, Wachsmuth R: Hyperactivity and parental psychopathology. J Child Psychol Psychiatry 31:381–392, 1990

Schachar R, Rutter M, Smith A: The characteristics of situationally and pervasively hyperactive children: implications for syndrome definition. J Child Psychol Psychiatry 22:375–392, 1981

Semrud-Clikeman MS, Biederman J, Sprich S, et al: Comorbidity between ADHD and learning disability: a review and report in a clinically referred sample. J Am Acad Child Adolesc Psychiatry 31:439–448, 1992

Silver LB: The relationship between learning disabilities, hyperactivity, distractibility, and behavioral problems. J Am Acad Child Psychiatry 20:385–397, 1981

Silver LB, Brunstetter RW: Attention deficit disorder in adolescents. Hosp Community Psychiatry 37:608–613, 1986

Spencer TJ, Biederman J, Wilens T, et al: Methylphenidate treatment in adults with childhood onset attention deficit hyperactivity disorder. Paper presented at the annual meeting of the American Academy of Child and Adolescent Psychiatry, Washington, DC, October 1992

Stewart MA, Morrison JR: Affective disorders among the relatives of hyperactive children. J Child Psychol Psychiatry 14:209–212, 1973

Stewart MA, deBlois CS, Cummings C: Psychiatric disorder in the parents of hyperactive boys and those with conduct disorder. J Child Psychol Psychiatry 21:283–292, 1980

Strober M, Morrell W, Burroughs J, et al: A family study of bipolar I disorder in adolescence: early onset of symptoms linked to increased familial loading and lithium resistance. J Affect Disord 15:255–268, 1988

Sylvester CE, Hyde TS, Reichler RJ: The Diagnostic Interview for Children and Personality Inventory for Children in studies of children at risk for anxiety disorders or depression. J Am Acad Child Adolesc Psychiatry 26:668–675, 1987

Szatmari P, Boyle M, Offord DR: ADDH and conduct disorder: degree of diagnostic overlap and differences among correlates. J Am Acad Child Adolesc Psychiatry 28:865–872, 1989

Tarter RE: Psychosocial history, minimal brain dysfunction and differential drinking patterns of male alcoholics. J Clin Psychol 38:867–873, 1982

Thorley G: Review of follow-up and follow-back studies of childhood hyperactivity. Psychol Bull 96:116–132, 1984

Wechsler D: Manual for the Wechsler Adult Intelligence Scale—Revised. San Antonio, TX, The Psychological Corporation, 1981

Weinberg WA, McLean A, Snider RL, et al: Depression, learning disability and school behavior problems. Psychol Rep 64:275–283, 1989

Weiss G: Follow up studies on outcome of hyperactive children. Psychopharmacol Bull 21:169–177, 1985

Weiss G, Hechtman LT: Hyperactive Children Grown Up. New York, Guilford, 1986

Weiss G, Hechtman L, Perlman T, et al: Hyperactives as young adults: a controlled prospective ten-year follow-up of 75 children. Arch Gen Psychiatry 36:675–681, 1979

Weiss G, Hechtman L, Milroy T, et al: Psychiatric status of hyperactives as adults: a controlled prospective 15-year follow-up of 63 hyperactive children. J Am Acad Child Psychiatry 24:211–220, 1985

Weissman MM, Gammon GD, John K, et al: Children of depressed parents: increased psychopathology and early onset of major depression. Arch Gen Psychiatry 44:847–853, 1987

Welner Z, Welner A, Stewart M, et al: A controlled study of siblings of hyperactive children. J Nerv Ment Dis 165:110–117, 1977

Wender PH, Reimherr FW, Wood DR, et al: Attention deficit disorder ("minimal brain dysfunction") in adults: a replication study of diagnosis and drug treatment. Arch Gen Psychiatry 38:449–456, 1981

Wender PH, Reimherr FW, Wood DR, et al: A controlled study of methylphenidate in the treatment of attention deficit disorder, residual type, in adults. Am J Psychiatry 142:547–552, 1985

Werry JS, Reeves JC, Elkind GS: Attention deficit, conduct, oppositional, and anxiety disorders in children, I: a review of research on differentiating characteristics. J Am Acad Child Adolesc Psychiatry 26:133–143, 1987

Wilens T, Biederman J: The stimulants, in Psychiatric Clinics of North America. Edited by Schaffer D. Philadelphia, PA, WB Saunders, 1992, pp 191–222

Wood DR, Reimherr FW, Wender PH, et al: Diagnosis and treatment of minimal brain dysfunction in adults: a preliminary report. Arch Gen Psychiatry 33:1453–1460, 1976

Wood DR, Wender PH, Reimherr FN, et al: The prevalence of attention deficit disorder, residual type, or minimal brain dysfunction, in a population of male alcoholic patients. Am J Psychiatry 140:95–98, 1983

Chapter 4

Conduct Disorder

**David R. Offord, M.D. and
Kathryn J. Bennett, M.Sc.**

T his chapter reviews the literature on conduct disorder in two areas, long-term outcome
and the effects of interventions. The review is
not intended to be exhaustive but its aim is to
summarize the major findings in these areas
and to suggest directions for future work.

▼ Long-Term Outcome

This section will cover the following topics:
continuity of aggression and violence, outcomes of conduct disorder, comorbidity, prognostic factors, causal mechanisms, and future
directions.

This chapter was originally published as Offord DR,
Bennett KJ: "Conduct Disorders: Long-Term Outcomes
and Intervention Effectiveness." *Journal of the American
Academy of Child and Adolescent Psychiatry* 33:1069–
1078, 1994. Used with permission. Copyright 1994
Williams & Wilkins.

Continuity of Aggression
and Violence

There is evidence from a number of studies that the stability of childhood-onset aggression during childhood and adolescence is considerable (Loeber 1982, 1991; Olweus 1979). Children who initially display high rates of antisocial behavior are more likely to continue in this behavior than children who initially show lower rates of antisocial behavior.

The Cambridge Study in Delinquent Development (Farrington 1991), a prospective longitudinal study of 411 males, provides data on this issue. The boys, who came from a working-class area in London, England, were first contacted in 1961 and 1962 when they were 8 years old. They were interviewed and tested in their schools when they were 8, 10, and 14 years of age, and the boys' teachers completed questionnaires when they were 8, 10, 12, and 14. The subjects were interviewed at ages 16, 18, 21, 25, and 32.

There was evidence of continuity of aggression and violence from ages 8–32. For example, children who were rated as aggressive by their teachers at ages 8–10 were significantly more likely to be rated as aggressive on the basis of self-reports at age 32, and to have been convicted of a violent crime sometime up to age 32. All measures of aggression and violence were significantly interrelated, showing that there was significant continuity in aggressiveness for ages 8–10 to age 32, and significant continuity from child aggressiveness to adult criminal violence. The strongest relationships were generally between the measures that were closest in time. Relationships over long periods of time were statistically significant but relatively weak. Further, aggression in childhood predicted later-life outcomes other than aggression and violence at age 32. These outcomes included unemployment, use of tobacco and illicit drugs, and driving while intoxicated. Lastly, all measures of youthful aggression were strongly related to chronic offending in young adults.

In summary, aggressive behavior in childhood predicts aggression in adolescence, and aggression in childhood and adolescence predicts aggression, violence, and other behaviors such as alcohol and substance abuse and chronic offending at age 32. The power of the prediction decreases as the time interval lengthens. All of these data, although anterospective in nature, apply to males only. There is a paucity of data on the outcome of aggressive behavior in girls.

Outcomes of Conduct Disorder

The studies that have addressed the issue of outcomes of conduct disorder can be categorized as outlined in Figure 4–1. The first division is between prospective and retrospective studies. Each of these categories can be further subdivided into studies that use a clinic or high-risk sample compared with those that use a community sample. Lastly, each of the resulting four categories can be subdivided into two groups: those studies that identify a group of children with conduct disorders who have been classified based on clinician input (CD symptoms group) and those studies in which the data on antisocial behavior in childhood and adolescence is expressed as symptom scores, or if a threshold or cutoff for conduct disorder has been set, no clinical input has been involved (AS symptoms group).

Examples of studies in Group A (prospective, clinic, or high-risk, CD) include a follow-up sample of Maudsley Hospital child psychiatric clinic attenders in 1968–1969 (Harrington et al. 1990, 1991) and a follow-up of children reared in group foster homes (Quinton

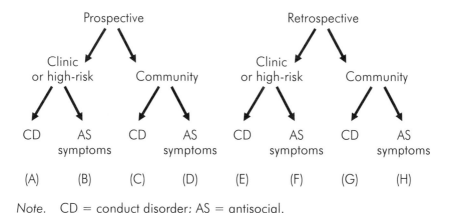

Note.   CD = conduct disorder; AS = antisocial.

Figure 4–1.   Types of studies examining the outcomes of conduct disorder.

and Rutter 1988; Rutter et al. 1990; Zoccolillo et al. 1992). These are not "real-time" prospective studies but involved the investigators making use of data already collected, when the sample was children and adolescents, and then collecting current data on them as adults. The limitation of these studies is that the samples are not representative of conduct disorder overall. They may, for example, include the more severe cases in which rates of comorbidity, in terms of the coexistence of other psychiatric disorders, is high, and in which the children and adolescents have grown up in surroundings of chronic psychosocial disadvantage. Some or all of these factors may have the effect of worsening the long-term outcome of conduct disorder.

A famous example of a study in Group B (prospective, clinic, or high-risk AS symptoms) is Robins' long-term follow-up of patients who attended the Municipal Child Guidance Clinic of St. Louis in the 1920s (Robins 1966). Here, the data available at the childhood level were contained in clinic and, in some cases, court records. Major findings from this study include the following: adults who qualified for a diagnosis of antisocial personality had almost all been antisocial as children; the variety of childhood antisocial behaviors was a better predictor of severe antisocial behavior than was any particular childhood behavior; and the child's own behavior was a better predictor of adult behavior than were family characteristics or social status. Lastly, children referred to the clinic for antisocial behavior had a much worse adult outcome than children referred for nonantisocial symptoms.

Examples of studies in Group C (prospective, community, CD) include the Ontario Child Health Study (OCHS) (Offord et al. 1992) and the Dunedin Multidisciplinary Health and Development Study (McGee et al. 1992). Both these studies used community samples and potentially have the ability to provide information on the outcome of conduct disorder in childhood and adolescence in a community sample in which clinician input has been present in classifying children as having conduct disorder or not. Unfortunately, the subjects in both of these studies are not old enough yet to provide information on the adult outcomes of conduct disorder. In the OCHS, the initial measures of conduct disorder are available from the first wave of data collection, which took place when the subjects were ages 4–12, and from the second wave, which took place when they were ages 8–16. The strongest predictor of conduct disorder in the second wave was the presence of conduct disorder 4 years earlier. More than 4 out of 10 children (44.8%), ages 4–12, classified as having conduct disorder in the 1983 OCHS, continued in that category at follow-up in 1987. Children originally classified as having conduct disorder also were categorized, in substantial proportions, in other diagnostic categories 4 years later—35.4% were hyperactive and 29.4% had emotional disorder. Somewhat less than half (46.1%) of children with conduct disorder fulfilled criteria 4 years later for one or more of the three aforementioned disorders. In the Dunedin birth cohort study, the children were classified psychiatrically by a clinician when they were 11 and 15 years of age. Externalizing disorder (conduct, oppositional, hyperactivity) at age 11 did not predict externalizing disorder at 15 for girls. However, for boys, externalizing disorder at age 11 strongly predicted externalizing disorder at age 15. These and similar studies should eventually contribute much-needed information on the adult outcomes of conduct disorder in a community sample.

An example of Group D (prospective, community AS symptoms) is the aforementioned Cambridge Study in Delinquent Development (Farrington 1991). This has been placed in the "community" category, although it could be argued that it should be placed in the "clinic or high-risk" category because the sample consisted of boys not from the community at large but from a working-class area. At the childhood level, no clinicians were involved in making the diagnosis of conduct disorder but rather reports of symptoms were obtained from multiple informants.

Now, proceeding to the studies using retrospective designs, there is none that has used clinicians to classify children as having conduct disorders based on retrospective data, that is, data that were gathered when they were adults. This would seem to be an impossible task. Thus, no studies exist in Groups E and G. Similarly, there are few or no relevant studies in Group F (retrospective, clinic, or high-risk, AS symptoms).

In contrast, there are several studies that can be classified in Group H (retrospective, community, AS symptoms). These include the study by Robins (1978) of young African American men whose names had been chosen from elementary school records and her study of Vietnam veterans. As with the Cambridge study, it could be argued that the study of young African American men, although a community sample, should be placed in the high-risk category. More recently, there is the Epidemiologic Catchment Area Study (ECA), which gathered data on approximately 20,000 adults 18 years and older in five sites in the United States (Robins and Regier 1991).

The studies that rely on retrospective self-reports have a number of limitations that could distort the accuracy of conclusions about the relationship between antisocial symptoms in childhood and adolescence and the adult outcome of conduct disorder (Robins and Price 1991). Two major ones will be mentioned. First, it may be that the willingness to admit symptoms at one point in life increases the willingness to admit symptoms at another point. Second, a survey of adults could not include those who died in childhood and early adolescence, a group that may be at increased risk for conduct disorder. Both of these factors could influence the results. In the first instance, the relationship between childhood antisocial behaviors and adult psychiatric symptoms may be enhanced whereas in the second, data would be missing on a group of children who have conduct disorders with a tragic early outcome.

A summary of this literature reveals that conduct problems predict antisocial behavior in adulthood. This prediction is stronger for males than for females. Conduct problems also predict alcohol abuse and dependence, and, more weakly, drug abuse and dependence, but again the predictive power is stronger in men than it is in women. However, conduct problems predict internalizing disorders more strongly in women than in men (Robins 1986). Thus, significant conduct problems in childhood predict the same increased rates of psychiatric disorder overall in men and in women but the patterns are different. Lastly, conduct problems predict in adulthood not just increased rates of psychiatric diagnoses, but also widespread social dysfunction.

Comorbidity

Comorbidity addresses the issue of the extent to which other co-existing symptoms or disorders in childhood make independent contributions to the adult outcome of conduct problems. Two disorders will be discussed briefly, hyperactivity and depression.

The Cambridge Study in Delinquent Development (Farrington et al. 1990) provides data addressing comorbid hyperactivity. These results suggest that the presence of hyperactivity in childhood coexisting with conduct problems predicts persistence of antisocial behavior at least at the juvenile level. However, the study has several limitations. The sample is a lower class, inner city one, and the measures of hyperactivity and conduct problems were not specifically designed with modern criteria in mind. The strengths of the study include its prospective longitudinal design, low attrition rate, and the multiple sources of data employed.

The results do give some support to the contention that the apparent relationship between hyperactivity in childhood and antisocial behavior in adulthood may be accounted for in large part by coexisting antisocial behavior at the childhood level (Lilienfeld and Waldman 1990). They also support the emerging finding from longitudinal studies that young children with antisocial and hyperactivity symptoms are a particularly high-risk group for later antisocial behavior (Moffit 1990).

In the case of depression coexisting with conduct disorder, evidence from the follow-up of Maudsley Hospital child psychiatric clinic attenders indicates that although child conduct disorder was associated with a much increased risk for adult criminality (assessed from official crime records), the risk was completely unaffected by the presence or absence of depression at the childhood level (Harrington et al. 1991; Rutter et al. 1994). Thus, although there is evidence that coexisting hyperactivity plays an independent role in predicting persistence of antisocial behavior at the juvenile level, this appears not to be true in the case of depression.

Prognostic Factors

A number of factors have been consistently associated with persistence of conduct disorder into adulthood. They include an unusually early age at onset, high rates of problem behaviors, a high variety of problem behaviors (e.g., theft and aggression), and behaviors displayed in multiple settings (e.g., home and school) (Loeber 1991). Low autonomic reactivity has also been associated with persistence (Magnusson et al. 1991; Raine et al. 1990), and hyperactivity, of course, may be a predictor of persistence.

Causal Mechanisms

Much work needs to be done to understand the mechanisms or developmental pathways by which conduct disorder proceeds to antisocial behavior in adulthood. These mechanisms will have to take into account the differences in outcome of conduct disorder in men and women, and include not only the occurrence of the central disorder but reactions of the people in the environment to it.

Future Directions

Prospective studies of community samples of children provide the best opportunity to understand more thoroughly the adult outcomes of conduct disorder. At the childhood level, psychometrically sound and clinically relevant measures of a wide variety of psychiatric disorders using data from different informants is a necessity. Measures of the sociodemographic and familial surroundings will also be needed. Data will have to be collected at regular intervals to allow the testing of hypothesized developmental pathways. At the adult level, data should be gathered not only on the psychiatric status of the grown-up sample but on their functioning in different domains of life. Such studies can give us more complete answers to the issue of meaningful thresholds for conduct disorder, the role of informants in the diagnosis, the role of comorbid psychiatric disorders, the role of sociodemographic and familial variables, and pathways by which children with conduct disorder proceed to poor or good outcomes in adulthood.

Lastly, there is enough known now to conclude that children with conduct disorder, as a group, have a poor adult outcome, and that individually based treatment is expensive and not very effective. Thus, there is a pressing need for prevention studies. If randomized controlled trials are used, the untreated group can provide the kind of information we need to enrich our understanding of the natural history of the disorder.

▼ Interventions and Their Effects

Is there evidence that the natural history of conduct disorder can be altered, thus avoiding the associated long-term negative outcomes? This section provides an overview of the effectiveness of four intervention strategies to prevent or treat conduct disorder: parent- and family-targeted programs, social-cognitive programs, peer- and school-based programs, and community programs.

Parent- and Family-Targeted Programs

Theoretical Base

Interventions that target parenting and family systems are based on a causal model wherein social interactional processes between the parent and child or within the family are thought to inadvertently develop and sustain aggressive and antisocial behavior (Patterson 1982, 1986; Patterson et al. 1982; Reid and Patterson 1991). Parent management training (PMT) is one of the most widely known familial interventions and aims to teach parents how to promote desirable, prosocial behaviors in their child while at the same time applying discipline to minimize undesirable, maladaptive behaviors.

Intervention Effectiveness

Substantial evidence regarding short-term effectiveness in clinical populations is available, including data collected in studies in which assignment to treatment was random (Kazdin 1987; Patterson et al. 1982). The body of available knowledge suggests that PMT holds promise, but a number of factors have been shown to moderate outcome, most notably parent characteristics and family social circumstances. Parent compliance in attending PMT is a serious problem. Some parents simply are not able to participate due to mental retardation, other psychopathology, substance abuse, or emotional crises caused by marital discord or family dysfunction (Kazdin

1987). Duration of treatment and therapist expertise have also been shown to influence treatment outcomes (Kazdin 1987).

Summary
The evidence regarding familial interventions is promising. However, most studies have been conducted under ideal conditions in clinical settings. Further studies with nonclinic populations are needed, including studies that assess the long-term impact of familial interventions, which has not been addressed in the studies to date. The major limitation is with respect to parent and family factors that moderate the impact of PMT, particularly parent compliance with the full regimen of sessions. Investigations that uncover ways to increase the motivation and ability of parents to participate will greatly enhance interventions for conduct disorder given the central etiological role of parents and family.

Social-Cognitive Programs

Theoretical Base
Social-cognitive interventions focus on the relationship between cognition and affect (thoughts and emotions) and behavior. The assumption is that changing or enhancing cognition and affect will lead to changed or enhanced behavioral adjustment. Deficits in problem-solving skills, perceptions, self-statements, and attributions have been shown to be associated with disruptive and antisocial behavior (Dodge 1986; Dodge and Frame 1982; Dodge and Newman 1981; Dodge et al. 1984; Kazdin 1990; Schneider 1989). Aggressive children are more likely to interpret the intentions and actions of others as hostile and to have poor social relations with peers, teachers, and parents. Aggressive children are also deficient with respect to their behavioral response repertoire (Dodge 1986; Schneider 1989). They identify fewer solutions to interpersonal problems and include physical force and aggression in their solutions more often when compared with nondisruptive children.

Intervention Effectiveness
A wide variety of intervention approaches has been developed, including problem-solving skills, anger control, coping skills, and

social skills. Training in problem-solving skills is derived from the work of Spivak and Shure (1974, 1976, 1978) and aims to teach five cognitive problem-solving skills on the assumption that these skills will lead to social competence and adjustment. Unfortunately, Spivak and Shure did not include blind outcome assessments in their studies of this approach, and no other investigator has been able to replicate their positive findings. Weissberg et al. (1991) designed a social problem-solving (SPS) program that focuses on developing social competence in young children in school settings using a variation on the Spivak and Shure approach. Their studies found a statistically significant improvement in SPS skills, but the relationship between SPS skills and improved adjustment was negative.

Anger coping and impulse control is another social-cognitive approach that uses problem solving and self-instruction to deal with anger-provoking situations or impulsive behavior (Kendall and Braswell 1982; Lochman and Curry 1986). Positive results on blind assessments of classroom and home behavior were found in studies conducted by these investigators.

Summary

The literature on the effectiveness of social-cognitive interventions is difficult to interpret due to the tremendous heterogeneity of children studied (e.g., adjusted versus maladjusted children, type and severity of preexisting behavioral disorder, and age group) as well as the range of intervention content and the instructional methods. A systematic review that categorizes studies according to these characteristics as well as the strength of the study design may reveal that the variation in findings can be explained substantially by specific features of the study design, study population, and the intervention under investigation.

Durlak (1985, 1991) has produced two extensive reviews of social-cognitive and cognitive-behavioral interventions, one using meta-analysis techniques. He concludes that the evidence for effectiveness is mixed and that the link between cognitive change and behavioral change has not been demonstrated. Other reviewers, including Ladd (1985), Schneider (1989), and Urbain and Kendall (1980), argue in favor of further experience and evaluation of these types of approaches.

Peer and School-Based Programs

Theoretical Base

The third class of intervention focuses on the role of peer relations and schools in the development of conduct disorder and antisocial behavior. Parental behavior may be the critical factor that leads to the development of undesirable behavior patterns during the preschool years. However, there is evidence that peer relations and school performance are the primary factors during middle childhood (DeV. Peters 1991; Eron et al. 1991).

It is argued that interventions that improve peer relations (usually through prosocial skills training) will reduce aggressive behavior and prevent the development of antisocial behavior. Up to 40% of rejected children are aggressive, and children who are aggressive and rejected have been shown to be at the highest risk to develop antisocial behavior in adolescence (Coie et al. 1991).

Interventions that target the school setting are derived from two bodies of literature. First, there is substantial evidence that school characteristics (such as the lack of a balance of high- and low-achieving students, poor classroom and school management techniques, and inadequate teaching practices) influence both academic achievement and behavior and that these effects are independent of student characteristics at school entry (Rutter 1983; Rutter et al. 1979). The second body of literature concerns the relationship between conduct disorder, poor academic achievement, and school failure (Hinshaw 1992; Schonfield et al. 1988). Hinshaw (1992) concluded in a comprehensive review that there is substantial evidence that academic and behavior problems are highly correlated. However, as the result of methodological weaknesses in the data, the evidence is insufficient to draw a firm conclusion about the direction of the relationship between academic problems and conduct disorder.

Intervention Effectiveness

Bierman and Furman (1984) and Bierman et al. (1987) developed a social-skills training program targeted at improving peer relations and acceptance. This approach focuses on skills acquisition and impact on aggressive behavior. Randomized studies conducted in primary-school boys rated to be highly aggressive and rejected were positive with respect to blind assessments of improved peer interaction and decreases in aggressive behavior.

Kellam et al. (1991) developed two interventions for classroomwide use in first grade called the Good Behavior Game and Mastery Learning. Both are applied by the teacher and aim to reduce levels of aggressive, disruptive, and shy behavior in the classroom and increase levels of reading achievement. Randomized studies of Mastery Learning in first-grade children have shown improvements in reading achievement. Similarly designed studies of the Good Behavior Game have shown improvements on unblinded measures of aggressive and shy behavior.

Two other early elementary school classroomwide approaches are worthy of mention (M. H. Boyle et al., unpublished observations, 1991; Reid and Patterson 1991). Large-scale trials are now underway in both Canada and the United States to evaluate the impact of school-based primary prevention programs offered to all children in the targeted grades. The programs target multiple systems—social skills and peer relations, parent and teacher management skills, academic skills, and recreational activities. Both initiatives are of great interest because they evaluate a systemwide primary prevention strategy offered universally to all children and involving teachers, parents, and peers.

Another strategy is the model presented by Comer (1980, 1985, 1988). This approach takes a systems perspective and aims to strengthen schools in socially disadvantaged communities through the establishment of a representative school governance and management group, a parent participation program, mental health teams, and curriculum development programs. The work was initiated in two extremely disadvantaged schools in New Haven in 1968. A comparison of 24 students from one of the experimental schools 3 years after completing the program with a similar number matched by age and sex who did not participate in the experimental schools showed the Comer program students were superior in terms of academic achievement and self-esteem. It is uncertain whether these differences are due to the program or to other differences between the two groups that could affect these outcomes (Comer 1985).

Summary

Evaluations of peer and school-based interventions are limited. The available studies provide little evidence for effectiveness on a population basis and do not address long-term outcomes. Only the reports of Boyle et al. (unpublished observations, 1991), Kellam et al. (1991), and Reid and Patterson (1991) address primary prevention, and all three projects are barely underway. The work by Bierman and Furman (1984), Bierman et al. (1987), and Coie et al. (1991) is suggestive of promising approaches for further testing. However, their interventions have been evaluated in extremely high-risk groups already experiencing significant behavior problems.

Community Programs

Theoretical Base

Community-based interventions for conduct disorder are either embedded in existing community-based programs or are the focus of new, specially targeted services at the community level. The goal is to strengthen the ability of the community to promote prosocial behavior and deter antisocial and delinquent behavior through changing or enhancing existing systems.

Intervention Effectiveness

The Cambridge-Somerville study is one of the earliest investigations of a community-based delinquency prevention program (McCord 1978; McCord and McCord 1959; Powers and Witmer 1951). The results of this study, which show that 30 years later the intervention group is worse off than the control group, are difficult to interpret. The 30-year follow-up data are of questionable validity due to a large sample loss, the potential for confounding, and the lack of random assignment of the original study groups.

Joffe and Offord (1987) reviewed 29 studies of prevention strategies conducted within the context of the community or specific community services, including vocational and recreational programs. Overall, very little evidence of effectiveness was found. However, the studies that employed stronger design methods tended to show positive results, particularly those that employed behavior modification techniques. An innovative, nonschool skill development program conducted in a publicly supported housing complex in Ottawa, Canada (Jones and Offord 1989; Offord and Jones 1983) showed statistically significant effects of antisocial behavior in community measures such as vandalism and police calls. However, no spillover effects on school performance were found at the end of the intervention period.

The role of early intervention through community-based primary prevention programs has recently been reviewed by Zigler et al. (1992). There is evidence that early intervention programs initiated in the 1960s and 1970s to enrich the preschool period and prevent school failure among high-risk populations have had an impact on delinquency and related behaviors. An example is the Perry Preschool Project (Berrueta-Clement et al. 1987), in which low-income, African American 3- and 4-year-old preschoolers at high risk for school failure were randomized to receive early childhood education, teacher home visits, and monthly parent-teacher small-group meetings, or no intervention. At age 19, children in the intervention group had higher secondary school graduation rates than children in the control group (67% vs. 49%). Only 31% of the intervention group had been arrested or charged compared with 51% of the control group. These impressive results must be interpreted in the context of the small sample size employed (n's are 58 and 65 for the intervention and nonintervention groups, respectively) and the population studied.

Summary

A number of promising approaches have been tried at the community level but there is little documented evidence of effectiveness. Community-based primary prevention programs should be given a high priority for several reasons. First, they can be made available to all children. This increases the likelihood of reaching every child who could benefit and minimizes the stigmatization and negative effects associated with labeling in a "high-risk" approach. Furthermore, including all children provides an opportunity for children with problems to interact with healthy peers in mixed gender settings. Evidence is available that low achievers and/or children with disruptive behavior do better when mixed with more well-adjusted children and that the presence of females in a group suppresses antisocial behavior in males (Offord 1989; Offord and Waters 1983). Community-based interventions can also include programs that are complementary to those offered through the medical, specialized mental health, and social service systems or the schools.

Future Directions

Overall, the available literature provides limited evidence for the effectiveness of either primary or secondary prevention. There is a great need to increase the scientific base for prevention and treatment interventions. Further studies should adhere to four key methodological standards. First, studies are needed in representative samples of children with, or at risk for, conduct disorder. Most of the currently available studies have been conducted in highly selected clinic samples of severely impaired children. The extent to which these findings can be generalized to populations of children at the community level is not clear. Second, rigorous randomized research designs that compare similar groups who receive or do not receive the intervention under investigation are needed to determine the benefit of promising interventions. Third, the intervention approach must be derived from empirically derived theories regarding the underlying mechanisms for conduct disorder and antisocial behavior. In addition, the intervention should be designed to ensure that it is feasible for implementation "in the real world" if the evaluation results are positive. The components of the intervention must be specified and operationalized in a manner that will allow others to reproduce it in their own settings, and there should be evidence that intervention integrity was achieved throughout the study. Fourth, the relevance of each measurement (or group of measures) selected to the hypothesized mechanism(s) of effect of the intervention must be explicitly addressed. The measures must be shown to have adequate reliability and validity (including sensitivity to change) in the population under investigation.

A final point concerns the need to conceptualize primary and secondary prevention for conduct disorder and antisocial behavior as an ongoing process that must begin in very early childhood and continue through adolescence and beyond. It is very unlikely that a time-limited intervention offered at one point in a child's life will permanently eliminate existing undesirable behaviors and/or protect against subsequent developmental or life stresses that occur after the intervention has ended.

▼ Conclusion

Conduct disorder constitutes a heavy burden of suffering in terms of its relatively high prevalence, its morbidity in childhood and beyond, and the extensive societal cost of the condition (Offord 1989). There are compelling arguments in favor of an increased emphasis on primary prevention efforts. These include the limited effectiveness of clinic-based treatment and the discrepancy that exists between the level of need that presently exists in the population and the limited resources available to treat individual children in a clinic setting. The payoff of discovering successful prevention programs for conduct disorder will not only be reduced levels of antisocial behavior in childhood and adolescence but lower frequencies of adult criminality and probably also of a wide array of psychosocial disturbances.

▼ References

Berrueta-Clement JR, Schweinhart LJ, Barnett WS, et al: The effects of early educational intervention on crime and delinquency in adolescence and early adulthood, in Primary Prevention of Psychopathology, Vol 10: Prevention of Delinquent Behaviour. Edited by Burchard JD, Burchard SN. Newbury Park, CA, Sage, 1987, pp 220–240

Bierman KL, Furman W: The effects of social skills training and peer involvement on the social adjustment of preadolescents. Child Dev 57:151–162, 1984

Bierman KL, Millar CL, Stabb SD: Improving the social behaviour and peer acceptance of rejected boys: effects of social skills training with instructions and prohibitions. J Consult Clin Psychol 55:194–200, 1987

Coie JD, Underwood M, Lochman JE: Programmatic intervention with aggressive children in the school setting, in The Development and Treatment of Childhood Aggression. Edited by Pepler DJ, Rubin KH. Hillsdale, NJ, Lawrence Erlbaum Associates, 1991, pp 389–410

Comer JP: School Power. New York, Free Press, 1980

Comer JP: The Yale-New Haven Primary Prevention Project: a follow-up study. J Am Acad Child Adolesc Psychiatry 24:154–160, 1985

Comer JP: Educating poor minority children. Sci Am 259:42–48, 1988

DeV Peters R: Expanding the perspective on contributing factors and service delivery approaches to childhood aggression, in The Development and Treatment of Childhood Aggression. Edited by Pepler DJ, Rubin KH. Hillsdale, NJ, Lawrence Erlbaum Associates, 1991, pp 189–197

Dodge KA: A social information processing model of social competence in children, in Minnesota Symposia on Child Psychology. Edited by Perlmutter M. Hillsdale, NJ, Lawrence Erlbaum Associates, 1986, pp 77–135

Dodge KA, Frame CL: Social cognitive biases and deficits in aggressive boys. Child Dev 51:620–635, 1982

Dodge KA, Newman JP: Biased decision-making processes in aggressive boys. J Abnorm Psychol 90:375–379, 1981

Dodge KA, Murphy RR, Buchsbaum K: The assessment of intention-cue detection skills in children: implications for developmental psychopathology. Child Dev 55:163–173, 1984

Durlak JA: Primary prevention of school maladjustment. J Consult Clin Psychol 53:623–630, 1985

Durlak JA: Effectiveness of cognitive-behaviour therapy for maladjusting children: a meta-analysis. Psychol Bull 110:204–214, 1991

Eron LD, Huesmann LR, Zelli A: The role of parental variables in the learning of aggression, in The Development and Treatment of Childhood Aggression. Edited by Pepler DJ, Rubin KH. Hillsdale, NJ, Lawrence Erlbaum Associates, 1991, pp 169–188

Farrington DP: Childhood aggression and adult violence: early precursors and later-life outcomes, in The Development and Treatment of Childhood Aggression. Edited by Pepler DJ, Rubin KH. Hillsdale, NJ, Lawrence Erlbaum Associates, 1991, pp 189–197

Farrington DP, Loeber R, Van Kammen WB: Long-term criminal outcomes of hyperactivity-impulsivity-attention deficit and conduct problems in childhood, in Straight and Devious Pathways from Childhood to Adulthood. Edited by Robins L, Rutter M. New York, Cambridge University Press, 1990, pp 62–81

Harrington R, Fudge H, Rutter M, et al: Adult outcomes of childhood and adolescent depression, I: psychiatric status. Arch Gen Psychiatry 47:465–473, 1990

Harrington R, Fudge H, Rutter M, et al: Adult outcome of childhood and adolescent depression, II: links with antisocial disorder. J Am Acad Child Adolesc Psychiatry 30:434–439, 1991

Hinshaw SP: Externalizing behavior problems and academic underachievement in childhood and adolescence: causal relationships and underlying mechanisms. Psychol Bull 111:127–155, 1992

Joffe RT, Offord DR: The primary prevention of antisocial behaviour. Journal of Preventive Psychiatry 3:251–259, 1987

Jones MB, Offord DR: Reduction of antisocial behavior in poor children by non-school skill development. J Child Psychol Psychiatry 30:737–750, 1989

Kazdin AE: Treatment of antisocial behavior in children: current status and future directions. Psychol Bull 102:187–203, 1987

Kazdin AE: Conduct disorders, in International Handbook of Behavior Modification and Therapy, 2nd Edition. Edited by Bellack AS, Hersen M, Kazdin AE. New York, Plenum, 1990, pp 669–707

Kellam SG, Werthamer-Larsson L, Dolan LJ, et al: Developmental epidemiologically based preventive trials: baseline modeling of early target behaviours and depressive symptoms. Am J Community Psychol 4:563–584, 1991

Kendall PC, Braswell L: Cognitive-behavioural self-control therapy for children: a components analysis. J Consult Clin Psychol 50:672–689, 1982

Ladd GW: Documenting the effects of social skill training with children: process and outcome assessment, in Children's Peer Relations: Issues in Assessment and Intervention. Edited by Schneider BH, Rubin KH, Ledingham JE. New York, Springer-Verlag New York, 1985, pp 243–269

Lilienfeld SO, Waldman ID: The relation between childhood attention-deficit hyperactivity disorder and adult antisocial behavior reexamined: the problem of heterogeneity. Clinical Psychology Review 10:699–725, 1990

Lochman JE, Curry JF: Effects of social problem-solving training and self-instruction training with aggressive boys. Journal of Clinical Child Psychology 15:159–164, 1986

Loeber R: The stability of antisocial and delinquent child behavior: a review. Child Dev 53:1431–1446, 1982

Loeber R: Antisocial behavior: more enduring than changeable? J Am Acad Child Adolesc Psychiatry 30:393–397, 1991

Magnusson D, Klinteberg B, Statton H: Autonomic activity/reactivity, behavior and crime in a longitudinal perspective. Report from the Department of Psychology, Stockholm University, No. 738, 1991

McCord J: A thirty-year follow-up of treatment effects. Am Psychol 33:284–289, 1978

McCord J, McCord NW: A follow-up report on the Cambridge-Somerville youth study. Annals of the American Academy of Political Sciences 322:89–96, 1959

McGee R, Feehan H, Williams S, et al: DSM-III disorders from age 11 to age 15. J Am Acad Child Adolesc Psychiatry 31:50–59, 1992

Moffit TE: Juvenile delinquency and attention deficit disorder: boys' developmental trajectories from age 3 to age 15. Child Dev 61:893–910, 1990

Offord DR: Conduct disorder: risk factors and prevention, in Prevention of Mental Disorders, Alcohol and Other Drug Use in Children and Adolescents (DHHS Publ No ADM 89-1646). Edited by Shaffer D, Philips I, Enzer NB. Washington, DC, Alcohol, Drug Use and Mental Health Administration, 1989, pp 273–307

Offord DR, Jones MB: Skill developent: a community intervention program for the prevention of antisocial behavior, in Childhood Psychopathology and Development. Edited by Guze SB, Earls FJ, Barrett JE. New York, Raven, 1983, pp 165–188

Offord DR, Waters BG: Socialization and its failure, in Developmental-Behavioral Pediatrics. Edited by Levine MD, Carey WB, Crocker AC, et al. Philadelphia, PA, WB Saunders, 1983, pp 650–682

Offord DR, Boyle MH, Racine YA, et al: Outcome, prognosis and risk in a longitudinal follow-up study. J Am Acad Child Adolesc Psychiatry 31:916–923, 1992

Olweus D: Stability of aggressive reaction patterns in males: a review. Psychol Bull 86:852–875, 1979

Patterson GR: Coercive Family Process. Eugene, OR, Castalia Publishing Co, 1982

Patterson GR: Performance models for antisocial boys. Am Psychol 41:432–444, 1986

Patterson GR, Chamberlain P, Reid JB: A comparative evaluation of a parent training program. Behavior Therapy 13:638–650, 1982

Powers E, Witmer H: An Experiment in the Prevention of Delinquency: The Cambridge-Somerville Youth Study. New York, Columbia University Press, 1951

Quinton D, Rutter M: Parenting Breakdown: The Making and Breaking of Inter-Generational Links. Avebury, England, Aldershot, 1988

Raine A, Venables PH, Williams M: Relationships between central and autonomic measures of arousal at age 15 years and criminality at age 24 years. Arch Gen Psychiatry 47:1003–1007, 1990

Reid JB, Patterson GR: Early prevention and intervention with conduct problems: a social interactional model for the integration of research and practice, in Interventions for Achievement and Behaviour Problems. Edited by Stoner G, Shinn MR, Walker HM. Silver Springs, MD, The National Association of School Psychologists, 1991, pp 715–739

Robins LN: Deviant Children Grown Up. Baltimore, MD, Williams & Wilkins, 1966

Robins LN: Sturdy childhood predictors of adult antisocial behavior: replications from longitudinal studies. Psychol Med 8:611–622, 1978

Robins LN: The consequences of conduct disorder in girls, in Development of Antisocial and Prosocial Behavior: Research, Theories and Issues. Edited by Olweus D, Block J, Radke-Yarrow M. New York, Academic Press, 1986, pp 385–414

Robins LN, Price RK: Adult disorders predicted by childhood conduct problems: results from the NIMH Epidemiologic Catchment Area Project. Psychiatry 54:116–132, 1991

Robins LN, Regier DA (ed): Psychiatric Disorders in America: The Epidemiologic Catchment Area Study. New York, The Free Press, 1991

Rutter M: School effects on pupil progress: research findings and policy implications. Child Dev 54:1–29, 1983

Rutter M, Maughan B, Mortimore P, et al: Fifteen Thousand Hours: Secondary Schools and Their Effects on Children. Cambridge, MA, Harvard University Press, 1979

Rutter M, Quinton D, Hill J: Adult outcomes of institution-reared children: males and females compared, in Straight and Devious Pathways from Childhood to Adulthood. Edited by Robins L, Rutter M. New York, Cambridge University Press, 1990, pp 135–157

Rutter M, Harrington R, Quinton D, et al: Adult outcomes of conduct disorder in childhood: implications for concepts and definitions of patterns of psychopathology, in Adolescent Problem Behaviors: Issues and Research. Edited by Ketterlinus RD, Lamb WE. Hillsdale, NJ, Lawrence Erlbaum and Associates, 1994, pp 57–80

Schneider BH: Between developmental wisdom and children's social-skills training, in Social Competence in Developmental Perspective. Edited by Schneider BH, Attili G, Weissberg RP. London, England, Kluwer Academic Publishers, 1989, pp 330–353

Schonfield IS, Shaffer D, O'Connor P, et al: Conduct disorder and cognitive functioning: testing three causal hypotheses. Child Dev 59:993–1007, 1988

Spivak G, Shure MB: Social Adjustment of Young Children: A Cognitive Approach to Solving Real-Life Problems. San Francisco, CA, Jossey-Bass, 1974

Spivak G, Shure MB: The Problem-Solving Approach to Adjustment. San Francisco, CA, Jossey-Bass, 1976

Spivak G, Shure MB: Problem Solving Techniques in Child-Rearing. San Francisco, CA, Jossey-Bass, 1978

Urbain ES, Kendall PC: Review of social-cognitive problem solving interventions with children. Psychol Bull 88:109–143, 1980

Weissberg RP, Caplan M, Harwood RL: Promoting competent young people in competence-enhancing environments: a systems-based perspective on primary prevention. J Consult Clin Psychol 59:830–841, 1991

Zigler E, Taussig C, Black K: Early childhood intervention: a promising preventative for juvenile delinquency. Am Psychol 47:997–1006, 1992

Zoccolillo M, Pickles A, Quinton D, et al: The outcome of conduct disorder: implications for defining adult personality disorder. Psychol Med 22:971–986, 1992

Chapter 5

Childhood Depression

**Valerie Del Medico, M.D.,
Elizabeth Weller, M.D., and
Ronald Weller, M.D.**

Knowledge of the long-term outcome of child and adolescent depressive disorders (dysthymia, major depression, and bipolar depression) is limited, but beginning to expand. Only within the past decade has depression in children and adolescents been recognized as a clinical phenomenon akin to adult depression with definite symptoms and natural history (Keller et al. 1988; Preskorn et al. 1987; Puig-Antich et al. 1978). In recent years depression in this age group has become a concern of organized psychiatry and a focus of research. For the clinician working with depressed youths and operating from a strong developmental perspective, concern about long-term outcome naturally arises. Fulfillment of a child or adolescent's personal potential and even survival to adulthood with an acceptable quality of life are at issue.

▼ Epidemiology

Depression in children and adolescents is now recognized as a significant public health problem. Estimates of the prevalence of depression in children and adolescents suggest that approximately 1% of preschoolers, 2% of school-age children, and 5% of adolescents are affected (Anderson et al. 1987; Kashani et al. 1987). Garrison et al. (1992) found a prevalence of major depression of approximately 9% in both males and females aged 12–14, and a prevalence of dysthymia of 8% in males and 5% in females. Their study utilized data from adolescents and their mothers. Epidemiological studies support the notion that the age at onset of first episode of mood disorder is becoming progressively younger, and incidence of affective disorder among more youthful cohorts is increasing (C. B. Burke et al. 1991; Gershon et al. 1987; Klerman 1988; Klerman and Weissman 1989). Greenberg et al. (1993) have pointed out that depression, because it begins to affect individuals at a relatively early age and is often not properly recognized, imposes a substantial burden on society.

The severity of depressive disorders in childhood and adolescence should not be underestimated. For example, psychosis is not uncommon in major depression that has a child or adolescent onset (Kovacs and Gastonis 1989; Strober and Carlson 1982). Substantial acute and long-term psychosocial impairment is seen in prepubertal-onset major depression (Puig-Antich et al. 1985a, 1985b). Likewise, the family dysfunction that has been noted during depressive episodes may persist despite remission of the depressive episode (Keitner and Miller 1990). In one prospective study (Geller et al. 1994), over 30% of 6- to 12-year-olds with major depression developed bipolar disorder when followed for 2–5 years.

From their survey of a large school-based sample of 15- and 16-year-olds, Kandel and Davies (1986) examined the sequelae of depressive symptoms with child and adolescent onsets. Dysphoria in adolescence predicted adult dysphoria. It also predicted psychiatric hospitalization, minor tranquilizer use in women, heavy cigarette smoking, delinquent or illegal activities, and accidents in men. Adolescent dysphoria was also associated with difficulty establishing close relationships with parents in adolescence and with spouses in young adulthood.

Teenage parenthood has been associated with depressive symptoms (Horowitz et al. 1991). Substance abuse, which is associated with both depression and suicide, has increased among adolescents in the United States (C. B. Burke et al. 1991). Suicide rates for adolescents 15–19 years of age have quadrupled in the past 40 years (Mortality and Morbidity Weekly Report 1991). Over 5,000 suicides per year occur in the 15- to 24-year-old age group, averaging 14 suicides daily. There are estimated to be five times as many suicide attempts as completed suicides in U.S. adolescents (Tishler et al. 1981). Suicides among 10- to 14-year-olds are responsible for approximately 560 deaths yearly (Hawton 1986).

▼ Delimitation, Episode Duration, and Recurrence

The need for appropriate and universal definitions of such terms as *remission, recovery, relapse,* and *recurrence* has only recently been recognized and addressed (Frank et al. 1991; Prien et al. 1991). Consistency of these terms must precede their operationalization to facilitate comparison of existing studies.

Do short-term factors such as symptom profile, index episode duration and severity, age at onset, or first recurrence predict long-term outcome? The literature on adult depression suggests that symptom severity and profile do affect episode duration (Keller et al. 1992), and that ongoing depressive symptoms may predict recurrence of major depression, as discussed subsequently. Although dysthymia and major depression are considered distinct disorders, this distinction may seem somewhat artificial at times. For example, many individuals who do not completely recover from a major depressive episode may continue in a dysthymic state (Keller et al. 1992) and subsyndromal depressive symptoms and/or dysthymia may predict major depression in adults (Horwath et al. 1992; Wells et al. 1992) and children (Warner et al. 1992). Kovacs et al. (1984) found that dysthymic disorder had an average duration of 3 years; and 89% of the 8- to 13-year-olds in their study who were diagnosed with dysthymia had recovered from the episode by 6.5 years. In the same study, the average length of a major depressive episode was

7.5 months and 72% of patients had suffered a recurrence at a 5-year follow-up. These observations are similar to those made by Asarnow et al. (1988) and Akiskal and Weller (1989). Fleming et al. (1993) found that approximately 25% of their depressed adolescents developed a serious major depression before a follow-up interview 4 years later. Garber et al. (1988) followed depressed adolescent psychiatric inpatients (mean age 14 years) for approximately 8 years after index admission. Seven of the 11 subjects had at least 1 episode of major depression. Of these, 4 had had more than 1 recurrence.

Most follow-up studies of depressed children and adolescents do not assess whether these subjects develop bipolar illness. However, the early age at onset of depression in bipolar individuals (Akiskal and Weller 1989) would suggest that this should be examined. Kovacs and Gastonis (1989) reported that 25% of depressed children had become manic when followed up as adolescents. Strober and Carlson (1982) reported that 28% of psychotic depressed adolescents experienced a manic episode at 2-year follow-up. In an extension of the study, Strober et al. (1993) noted that time to recovery did not vary between psychotic and nonpsychotic depressed patients. Manic switching was observed only among psychotic subjects. Usefulness of psychotic depression as a prognosticator of bipolar illness may have been underestimated because of the briefness of the follow-up. These findings have important clinical ramifications in terms of diagnosis, treatment, and psychoeducation of youths with a history of psychotic depression and their families.

▼ Research Difficulties

Factors complicating research on long-term outcome in depression are many. They extend beyond the typical difficulty of conducting prospective, rater-blind studies on sufficient numbers of subjects using adequate outcome measures. The determination of adequate follow-up time, for example, is an important consideration. Only recently have prospective and retrospective studies yielded some useful guidelines suggesting 2 years or longer.

Diagnostic considerations are also an issue, particularly consistent standards of "caseness" at initial episode. As mentioned in the preceding section, distinctions between diagnoses may seem somewhat artificial at times. Clinical samples are also rife with comorbidity, and the role played by the amount and type of comorbidity in outcome is still not well defined. Some studies addressing comorbidity and follow-up will be presented later.

Even more difficult to determine and of immediate clinical importance are demographic and psychosocial features of subject history that appear to improve resiliency or vulnerability with respect to negative outcome. Some family studies may offer insights into these issues.

Finally, there is the role of treatment in long-term outcome of depressive disorders. Well-designed studies of both short-term and maintenance treatment are needed to address this issue.

Conners (1992) noted that extant studies of pharmacotherapy in adolescent depression generally did not examine behavioral, social, or academic variables that clinicians use to assess antidepressant efficacy. Duration of follow-up is also frequently insufficient in these studies for both short- and long-term assessment. This issue has also been examined in the adult literature (Quitkin et al. 1986). Furthermore, medication studies should consistently use and report blood levels and dosage per weight. Other difficulties include patient characterization and the apparently high incidence of bipolar outcome in early-onset major depression. We do not know the impact of initial pharmacotherapy on eventual course in these individuals.

Studies of the impact of nonpharmacological interventions on long-term outcome with adequate follow-up time are also scarce. More well-designed studies of this nature will be available as advances in operationalization in shorter term studies are made. The situation becomes even more complex when studies comparing the effects of psychotherapy and pharmacotherapy versus a combination of the two are attempted (Conte et al. 1986). Sometimes vaguely defined treater-patient interactions are considered the "placebo" for therapy.

▼ Prospective Studies

Giaconia et al. (1994) found that when onset of psychiatric disorders, including major depression, occurred before age 14, the risk of co-occurring disorders was increased. Coryell et al. (1991) noted that youth and a history of nonaffective illness are important risk factors for the recurrence of major affective disorders in adulthood.

Smith and Steiner (1992) found that girls with concurrent anorexia nervosa and major depression showed greater psychopathology and reported more depressive symptoms at 2-year follow-up than did those with anorexia alone. At diagnosis, however, girls with both conditions did not show more severe anorexic symptomatology than did those with anorexia nervosa alone. Hall et al. (1984) noted that comorbid dysthymia and anorexia nervosa had a similar relationship.

Wenning et al. (1993) have provided a preliminary examination of the relationship between oppositional defiant disorder and mood disorders. They studied a group of 28 latency-age children diagnosed with oppositional defiant disorder. Half of their outpatient sample met criteria for dysthymia. Kovacs et al. (1988) found a 25% comorbidity of mood disorder and conduct disorder in their sample of depressed children. Other studies have found a comorbidity near 35% for these two disorders (Kashani et al. 1987; Marriage et al. 1986; Puig-Antich 1982). Harrington et al. (1991), in their follow-up of juvenile patients into adulthood, found that outcomes of those with conduct disorder accompanying index depression were very similar to outcomes of nondepressed children with conduct disorder. There was also a strong trend for depressed individuals with conduct disorder to have a *higher* risk of adult depression than their nondepressed counterparts. Depressed subjects with conduct disorder had a worse short-term outcome and a higher risk of adult criminality.

Zoccolillo and Rogers (1992) followed adolescent girls with conduct disorder after psychiatric hospitalization, reevaluating them at 2–4 years. The majority also had depressive or anxiety disorders. Most of the girls dropped out of school, half were arrested, and one-third were pregnant before age 17. Many suffered traumatic injuries and 6% had died a violent death.

Keller et al. (1992) found high comorbidity of depression and anxiety disorders in their nonclinical sample of children and adolescents. McCauley et al. (1993) found comorbid anxiety disorder significantly related to severity of index depression. Strauss et al. (1988) studied children and adolescents referred for outpatient treatment of anxiety disorders. Twenty-eight percent of patients with anxiety disorder as diagnosed by DSM-III (American Psychiatric Association 1980) had concurrent major depression. These children were older, had more anxiety symptoms, and had a preponderance of certain anxiety disorders. Comorbidity of panic disorder and major depression or dysthymia has been described (Alessi and Magen 1988). More long-term follow-up studies on these anxious and depressed children are needed.

One study that followed patients with pediatric obsessive-compulsive disorder (OCD) 2–7 years after their initial presentation found that 68% still had OCD, and 12% had an additional diagnosis of depression or another anxiety disorder.

Substance abuse has been frequently found to be comorbid with depression (Deykin et al. 1992; Famularo et al. 1985; Kashani et al. 1985). The study by Deykin et al. (1992) suggests that there are several subgroups of adolescents with comorbid substance abuse, only one of which is a true dual diagnosis group. Further studies addressing long-term outcome within these subgroups should be undertaken.

▼ Family Studies

An association between family dysfunction and depressive disorders has been documented (Bird et al. 1988; Garrison et al. 1986; Kandel and Davies 1986; Kashani et al. 1985). Asarnow et al. (1993) found persistent mood disorder at 1-year posthospitalization follow-up among depressed children returning to homes in which family members were rated high on expressed emotion (EE). In a study by Warner et al. (1992), multiple parental depressive episodes or parental divorce was associated with a more protracted episode of major depression in children. Keller et al. (1986) also reported that the characteristics of parental psychiatric illness had important effects on their children. Parker and Hadzi-Pavlovic (1992) found that "anomalous parenting" as measured by the Parental Bonding Instrument (PBI) increased the risk of nonmelancholic depression in children. A "low parental care" rating on the PBI predicted the highest risk. In a study by McCauley et al.

(1993), family stress in the environment was the only predictor significantly related to overall psychosocial competence in depressed children over 3-year follow-up.

Hughes et al. (1992) divided adult subjects into three groups based on family history of depression. The pure depressive disease (PDD) group consisted of first-degree relatives with depression but no other psychiatric disorder. The depressive spectrum disease (DSD) group was generally a late-onset subtype with no family history of psychiatric disorder. The sporadic depressive disease group (SDD) reported no history of psychiatric disorders in first-degree relatives. Subjects in the DSD group experienced the most episodes of depression, followed in order by those in the SDD and PDD group. Low self-confidence was associated with more baseline depressive symptoms. Low self-confidence was not associated with outcome in PDD or SDD subjects. Severity of depression in SDD subjects was associated with low self-confidence. The authors postulated that PDD individuals have the advantage of some previous exposure to depression through their relatives. Subjects in the DSD group with high self-confidence fared worse in terms of course of depression. The authors felt this finding might be due to aggressive and self-centered character traits leading to a more characterological type of depression. These findings suggest that self-confidence has a protective effect against depression only in certain family history–based subtypes.

Several studies have associated low self-esteem with increased risk for depressive disorders (Kashani et al. 1983; Williams et al. 1989). It is not clear whether low self-esteem is a prodromal symptom of depression, a residual symptom of an unidentified previous episode, a personality trait resulting in vulnerability to depression, or a consequence of family dysfunction. Furthermore, it is not known if low self-esteem is related to decreased personal efficacy secondary to depression and/or failure to achieve developmental milestones.

R. J. Burke and Weir (1978) and D'Arcy and Siddique (1984) explained the increased occurrence of depression observed in female adolescents by higher stress and lower levels of mastery and self-esteem in this group. Recent work by Avison and McAlpine (1992) also supports this view. Rates of prepubertal depression appear to be roughly equal in males and females, with the girl–boy ratio increasing with age (Kashani et al. 1987). These studies suggested that gender socialization may play a role in the progressive excess of depression in females with increasing age.

Fleming and Offord (1990) critically reviewed the methodology and results of 14 epidemiological studies of child and adolescent depressive disorders. As part of their review, they summarized the reported prevalence, comorbidity, risk factors, and outcome. They specifically noted significant association of depressive disorders with family dysfunction and low self-esteem, which merit examination as prognostic factors.

Stressful life events in youth occur in a family context, and have been associated both with adult and with juvenile depression (Brown et al. 1977). A study by Bird et al. (1989) showed significant association between stressful life events and depression in youth. Parental loss either through death or separation (Adam et al. 1982; Brown et al. 1977) has been a stressful event of great prognostic interest.

Duggan et al. (1991) recontacted a series of consecutive inpatients (ages 16–67 at initial admission) more than 18 years after their index admissions. All met Research Diagnostic Criteria for major depression. Severe dysphoria, past history of alcoholism, separation from a parent, and chronic physical illness were most predictive of suicide attempts. Severe dysphoria and separation from a parent other than by death before age 17 were most strongly associated with frequency of suicide attempts, but not with medical severity of attempt.

Weller et al. (1991) found that recently bereaved prepubertal children endorsed many depressive symptoms and 37% met DSM-III-R (American Psychiatric Association 1987) symptom criteria for a major depressive episode. Risk factors for depression in bereaved children included previous history of depression, family history of depression, and increased stress after the bereavement.

Stressful life events have been associated with depression reported by the child but not identified by the parent (Costello et al. 1988). Such agents have also been associated with depression for white but not African American adolescents (Garrison et al. 1986). Hammen et al. (1988) found that initial depressive symptoms and life stress, but not attributions, for negative outcomes predicted the development of depression in children. However, neither attributions for negative outcomes nor interaction of attributions was predicted by stressful life events.

▼ Treatment

Potential treatment modalities in child and adolescent depressive disorders include individual, group, and family psychotherapy; play therapy; parent training; remedial education; out-of-home placement; and pharmacotherapy. Before initiation of any treatment, a comprehensive diagnostic evaluation synthesizing information from school, family, and patient is required. Because many parents may not be fully aware of or may not understand the inner life of their children, proper use of multiple sources of information is critical to obtaining an accurate symptom profile (Barrett et al. 1991). For example, adolescents may be particularly resistant to revealing private feelings. Prepubertal children may be unable to provide fully accurate and chronologically correct information.

A thorough physical exam including vital signs, growth chart completion, EKG and lab studies, and diagnostics as indicated are needed to rule out organic causes of mood symptoms and to obtain baseline data before initiation of pharmacotherapy. If pharmacotherapy is considered, drug choice, side effects, and use of plasma drug level monitoring should be carefully considered. In general, gradual dosage increases, use of minimum effective dosage, and avoidance of polypharmacy are desirable.

Outcome

Assessment of the effects of group, individual, and family therapy is complicated by the lack of a standardized approach to assessment and the lack of consensus on relevant outcome measures. Studies of individual psychotherapy in depressed juveniles are relatively scarce (Bemporad 1988). Several well-controlled studies of psychotherapy and family therapy have not determined their effectiveness (McConville and Bruce 1985; Puig-Antich and Gittelman 1982).

Taylor and McLean (1993) found that the majority of their adult patients, regardless of treatment type (behavior therapy, amitriptyline, psychodynamic psychotherapy, or relaxation) experienced either recovery or nonremission, with relatively few occurrences of remission followed by recurrence at 3-month follow-up. Nonremission profiles were characterized by a longer and more severe index episode and more personality disturbance. Predictors of vulnerability to depression such as sex, marital status, and family history of depression did not differ between responders and nonresponders. Although theirs was a short-term study focusing on treatment outcome, the findings are thought provoking. Could childhood interventions that ameliorate disturbance of the developing personality improve resilience against adult recurrences? Several studies have shown positive effects for therapeutic support groups, skills training, or relaxation training administered according to a standardized therapy manual (Fine et al. 1991; Reynolds and Coats 1986). Unfortunately, follow-up period was at less than 1 year and diagnostic criteria were not stringent.

Studies on the efficacy of tricyclic antidepressants have been somewhat equivocal (Kramer and Feiguine 1983; Kutcher et al. 1989; LaPierre and Raval 1984; Ryan et al 1986). Recent studies have underlined the importance of monitoring plasma concentration of tricyclic antidepressants (TCAs) (Geller et al. 1986; Preskorn et al. 1982; Puig-Antich et al. 1978). Unfortunately, most of the abovementioned studies had small sample sizes. Preskorn et al. (1982) obtained a 92% response rate with adequate plasma TCA concentration in 12 children who had not responded to 2 weeks of psychotherapy. The 7-year follow-up reported 80% drug response versus 20% placebo response (Preskorn et al. 1987). However, Geller et al. (1989) did not find a significant difference in response in depressed children treated with nortriptyline compared with control subjects, even with an adequate plasma level of nortriptyline. Hughes et al. (1990) have pointed out the importance of comorbidity subgrouping in terms of assessing medication response rate.

Most depressed individuals in the United States are untreated or are inappropriately treated (Keller et al. 1982, 1986). Brumback and Weinberg (1991) make a case for adequate pharmacotherapy and psychosocial intervention in depressed children and adoles-

Asarnow JR, Goldstein MJ, Carlson GA, et al: Childhood onset depressive disorders: a follow-up study on rates of rehospitalizations and out of home placement among child psychiatric inpatients. J Affect Disord 15:245–253, 1988

Asarnow JR, Goldstein MJ, Tompson M, et al: One year outcomes of depressive disorders in child psychiatric in-patients: evaluation of the prognostic power of a brief measure of expressed emotion. J Child Psychol Psychiatry 34:129–137, 1993

Avison WR, McAlpine DD: Gender difference in symptoms of depression among adolescents. J Health Soc Behav 33:77–96, 1992

Barrett ML, Berney TP, Bhake S, et al: Diagnosing childhood depression: who should be interviewed—parent or child? Br J Psychiatry 159 (suppl 11):22–27, 1991

Bemporad J: Psychodynamic treatment of depressed adolescents. J Clin Psychiatry 49:26–34, 1988

Bird HR, Canino G, Rubio-Stipee M, et al: Estimate of the prevalence of childhood maladjustment in a community survey in Puerto Rico. Arch Gen Psychiatry 45:1120–1126, 1988

Bird HR, Gould MS, Yager T, et al: Risk factors for maladjustment in Puerto Rican children. J Am Acad Child Adolesc Psychiatry 28:847–850, 1989

Brown GW, Harris T, Copeland JR: Depression and loss. Br J Psychiatry 130:1–18, 1977

Brumback RA, Weinberg WA: Pediatric behavioral neurology: an update on the neurologic aspects of depression, hyperactivity, and learning disabilities. Neurol Clin 8:677–703, 1991

Burke CB, Burke JD, Rae DS, et al: Comparing age at onset of major depression and other psychiatric disorders by birth cohorts in five U.S. community populations. Arch Gen Psychiatry 48:789–795, 1991

Burke RJ, Weir T: Differences in adolescent life stress, social support and well being. J Psychol 98:277–288, 1978

Conners CK: Methodology of antidepressant drug trials for treating depression in adolescents. Journal of Child and Adolescent Psychopharmacology 2:11–22, 1992

Conte HR, Plutchik R, Wild R, et al: Combined psychotherapy and pharmacotherapy for depression. Arch Gen Psychiatry 43:471–479, 1986

Coryell W, Endicott J, Keller MB: Predictors of relapse into major depressive disorder in a non-clinical population. Am J Psychiatry 148:1353–1358, 1991

Costello EJ, Edelbrock C, Burns BJ, et al: Psychiatric disorders in pediatric primary care. Arch Gen Psychiatry 45:1107–1116, 1988

D'Arcy C, Siddique CM: Psychological distress among Canadian adolescents. Psychol Med 14:615–625, 1984

Deykin EY, Buka SL, Zeena TH: Depressive illness among chemically dependent adolescents. Am J Psychiatry 149:1341–1347, 1992

Famularo R, Stone K, Popper C: Preadolescent alcohol abuse and dependence. Am J Psychiatry 140:1187–1189, 1985

Fine S, Forth A, Gilbert M, et al: Group therapy for adolescent depressive disorder: a comparison of social skills and therapeutic support. J Am Acad Child Adolesc Psychiatry 30:79–85, 1991

Fleming JE, Offord DR: Epidemiology of childhood depressive disorders: a critical review. J Am Acad Child Adolesc Psychiatry 29:571–580, 1990

Fleming JE, Boyle MH, Offord DR: The outcome of adolescent depression in the Ontario Child Health Study follow-up. J Am Acad Child Adolesc Psychiatry 32:28–33, 1993

Frank E, Prien RF, Jarrett RB, et al: Conceptualization and rationale for consensus definitions of terms in major depressive disorder: remission, recovery, relapse and recurrence. Arch Gen Psychiatry 48:851–855, 1991

Garber J, Kriss MR, Koch M, et al: Recurrent depression in adolescents: a follow-up study. J Am Acad Child Adolesc Psychiatry 27:49–54, 1988

Garrison CZ, Schluchter MD, Schoenback VJ, et al: Epidemiology of depressive symptoms in young adolescents. J Am Acad Child Adolesc Psychiatry 29:571–580, 1986.

Garrison CZ, Addy CL, Jackson KL, et al: Major depressive disorder and dysthymia in young adolescents. Am J Epidemiol 135:792–802, 1992

Geller B, Cooper TB, Chestnut EC, et al: Preliminary data on the relationship between nortriptyline plasma level and response in depressed children. Am J Psychiatry 143:1283–1286, 1986

Geller B, Cooper TB, McCombs HG, et al: Double blind placebo controlled study of nortriptyline in depressed children using a "fixed plasma level" design. Psychopharmacol Bull 25:101–108, 1989

Gershon ES, Hamovit JH, Guroff JJ, et al: Birth cohort analysis of secular trends in manic and depressive disorders in relatives of bipolar and schizoaffective patients. Arch Gen Psychiatry 44: 314–319, 1987

Giaconia RM, Reinherz HZ, Silverman AB, et al: Age of onset of psychiatric disorders in a community sample of older adolescents. J Am Acad Child Adolesc Psychiatry 33:706–717, 1994

Greenberg PE, Stiglin LE, Finkelstein SN, et al: Depression: a neglected major illness. J Clin Psychiatry 54:419–424, 1993

Hall A, Slim E, Hawker F, et al: Anorexia nervosa: long term outcome in 50 female patients. Br J Psychiatry 145:407–413, 1984

Hammen C, Adnan C, Hiroto D: A longitudinal study of diagnoses in children of women with unipolar and bipolar affective disorder. Arch Gen Psychiatry 47:1112–1117, 1988

Harrington R, Fudge H, Rutter M, et al: Adult outcomes of childhood and adolescent depression, II: links with antisocial disorders. J Am Acad Child Adolesc Psychiatry 30:434–439, 1991

Hawton K: Suicide and Attempted Suicide Among Adolescents. Beverly Hills, CA, Sage, 1986

Horowitz SM, Klerman LV, Kuo HS, et al: Intergenerational transmission of school-age parenthood. Family Planning Perspectives 23:168–172, 1991

Horwath E, Johnson J, Klerman GI, et al: Depressive symptoms as relative and attributable risk factors for first onset major depression. Arch Gen Psychiatry 49:817–823, 1992

Hughes C, Preskorn S, Weller EB, et al: The effect of concomitant disorders in childhood depression on predicting treatment response. Psychopharmacol Bull 26:235–238, 1990

Hughes DC, Turnbull JE , Blazer DG: Family history of psychiatric disorder and low self-confidence: predictors of depressive symptoms at 12 month follow up. J Affect Disord 25:197–212, 1992

Kandel DB, Davies M: Adult sequelae of adolescent depressive symptoms. Arch Gen Psychiatry 43:255–262, 1986

Kashani JH, Henrichs TF, Reid JC, et al: Depression in diagnostic subtypes of delinquent boys. Adolescence 17:943–949, 1982

Kashani JH, McGee R, Carlson S, et al: Depression in a sample of 9 year old children: prevalence and associated characteristics. Arch Gen Psychiatry 40:1217–1223, 1983

Kashani JH, Keller MB, Soloman N, et al: Double depression in adolescent substance abusers. J Affect Disord 8:153–157, 1985

Kashani JH, Carlson GA, Beck NC, et al: Depression, depressive symptoms and depressed mood among a community sample of adolescents. Am J Psychiatry 144:931–934, 1987

Keitner GI , Miller IW: Family functioning and major depression: an overview. Am J Psychiatry 147:1128–1137, 1990

Keller MB, Klerman GL, Lavori PW, et al: Treatment received by depressed patients. JAMA 248:1848–1855, 1982

Keller MB, Beardslee WR, Dorer DJ, et al: Impact of severity and chronicity of parental affective illness on adaptive functioning and psychopathology in children. Arch Gen Psychiatry 43:930–937, 1986

Keller MB, Beardslee W, Lavori PW, et al: Course of major depression in non-referred adolescents: a retrospective study. J Affect Disord 15:235–243, 1988

Keller MB, Lavori PW, Beardslee WR, et al: Depression in children and adolescents: new data on "undertreatment" and a literature review on the efficacy of available treatments. J Affect Disord 21:163–171, 1991

Keller MB, Lavori PW, Mueller TI, et al: Time to recovery, chronicity, and levels of psychopathology in major depression: a five year prospective follow up of 431 subjects. Arch Gen Psychiatry 49:809–816, 1992

Klerman GL: The current age of youthful melancholia: evidence for increase in depression among adolescents and young adults. Br J Psychiatry 152:4–14, 1988

Klerman GL, Weissman MM: Increasing rates of depression. JAMA 261:2229–2235, 1989

Kovacs M, Gastonis C: Stability and change in childhood onset depressive disorders: longitudinal course as a diagnostic validator, in The Validity of Psychiatric Diagnosis. Edited by Robins LN, Barrett JE. New York, Raven, 1989, pp 57–76

Kovacs M, Feinberg T, Croose-Novak M, et al: Depressive disorders in children, II: a longitudinal study of the risk for subsequent major depression. Arch Gen Psychiatry 41:643–649, 1984

Kovacs M, Paulauskas S, Gastonis C, et al: Depressive disorders in childhood, III: a longitudinal study of comorbidity with a risk for conduct disorders. J Affect Disord 15:205–217, 1988

Kramer AD, Feiguine RJ: Clinical effects of amitriptyline in adolescent depression: a pilot study. J Am Acad Child Adolesc Psychiatry 20:636–644, 1983

Kutcher SP, Marton P, Korenblum M: Relationship between psychiatric illness and conduct disorder in adolescents. Can J Psychiatry 34:526–529, 1989

LaPierre YD, Raval KJ: Pharmacotherapy of affective disorders in children and adolescents. Psychiatr Clin North Am 12:951–961, 1984

Marriage K, Fine S, Moretti, et al: Relationship between depression and conduct disorder in children and adolescents. J Am Acad Child Adolesc Psychiatry 25:687–691, 1986

McCauley E, Myers K, Mitchell J, et al: Depression in young people: initial presentation and clinical course. J Am Acad Child Adolesc Psychiatry 32:714–722, 1993

McConville BJ, Bruce RT: Depressive illness in children and adolescents: a review of current concepts. Can J Psychiatry 30:119–129, 1985

Mortality and Morbidity Weekly Report: Attempted suicide among high school students—United States. Mortality and Morbidity Weekly Report 40:633–635, 1991

Parker G, Hadzi-Pavlovic D: Parental representations of melancholic and nonmelancholic depressives: examining for specificity to depressive type and for evidence of additive effects. Psychol Med 22:657–665, 1992

Preskorn SH, Weller EB, Weller RA: Depression in children: relationship between plasma imipramine levels and response. J Clin Psychiatry 43:450–453, 1982

Preskorn SK, Weller EB, Weller RA, et al: Depression in prepubertal children: dexamethasone nonsuppression predicts differential responses to imipramine vs placebo. Psychopharmacol Bull 23:128–133, 1987

Prien RF, Carpenter LL, Kupfer DJ: The definition and operational criteria for treatment outcome of major depressive disorder: a review of the current literature. Arch Gen Psychiatry 48:796–800, 1991

Puig-Antich J: Major depression and conduct disorder in puberty. J Am Acad Child Adolesc Psychiatry 21:118–128, 1982

Puig-Antich J, Gittelman R: Depression in childhood and adolescence, in Handbook of Affect Disorders. Edited by Paykel ES. New York, Guilford, 1982, pp 379–392

Puig-Antich J, Blau S, Marx N, et al: Prepubertal major depressive disorder: a pilot study. J Am Acad Child Adolesc Psychiatry 17:695–707, 1978

Puig-Antich J, Lukens E, Davies M, et al: Psychosocial functioning in prepubertal MD disorders, I: interpersonal relationships during the depressive episode. Arch Gen Psychiatry 42:500–507, 1985a

Puig-Antich J, Lukens E, Davies M, et al: Psychosocial functioning in prepubertal MD disorders, II: interpersonal relationships after sustained recovery from the depressive episode. Arch Gen Psychiatry 42:511–517, 1985b

Quitkin F, Rabkin J, Stewart J, et al: Study duration in antidepressant research: advantage of a 12 week trial. J Psychiatr Res 20:211–216, 1986

Reynolds WM, Coats KJ: A comparison of cognitive-behavioral therapy and relaxation training for the treatment of depression in adolescents. J Consult Clin Psychol 54:653–660, 1986

Ryan N, Puig-Antich J, Cooper T, et al: Imipramine in adolescent major depression: plasma levels and clinical response. Acta Psychiatr Scand 73:275–288, 1986

Smith C, Steiner H: Psychopathology in anorexia nervosa and depression. J Am Acad Child Adolesc Psychiatry 31:841–843, 1992

Strauss CC, Last CG, Hersen M, et al: Association between anxiety and depression in children and adolescents with anxiety disorders. J Abnorm Child Psychol 16:57–68, 1988

Strober M, Carlson G: Predictors of bipolar illness in adolescents with major depression: a follow up investigation. Adolesc Psychiatry 10:299–319, 1982

Strober M, Lampert C, Schmidt S, et al: The course of major depressive disorder in adolescents, I: recovery and risk of manic switching in a follow-up of psychotic and nonpsychotic subtypes. J Am Acad Child Adolesc Psychiatry 32:34–43, 1993

Taylor S, McLean P: Outcome profiles in the treatment of unipolar depression. Behav Res Ther 31:325–330, 1993

Tishler CL, McKenry PC, Morgan KC: Adolescent suicide attempts: some significant factors. Suicide Life Threat Behav 11:86–92, 1981

Warner V, Weissman MM, Fendrech M, et al.: The course of major depression in the offspring of depressed parents: incidence, recurrence and recovery. Arch Gen Psychiatry 49:795–801, 1992

Weller EB, Weller RA, Fristad MA, et al: Depression in recently bereaved prepubertal children. Am J Psychiatry 148:36–40, 1991

Wells KB, Burnham MA , Rogers W: Course of depression for adult outpatients: results from the medical study. Arch Gen Psychiatry 49:788–794, 1992

Weinberg WA, McLean A, Snider RL, et al: Depression, learning disability, and school behavior problems. Psychol Rep 64:275–283

Wenning K, Nathan P, King S: Mood disorders in children with oppositional defiant disorder: a pilot study. Am J Orthopsychiatry 63:295–299, 1993

Williams S, McGee R, Anderson J, et al: The structure and correlates of self-reported symptoms in 11 year old children. J Abnorm Child Psychol 17:55–71, 1989

Zoccolillo M, Rogers K: Characteristics and outcome of hospitalized adolescent girls with conduct disorder. J Am Acad Child Adolesc Psychiatry 30:973–981, 1991

Chapter 6

Suicidal Behavior

Cynthia R. Pfeffer, M.D.

Since the late 1960s, the rates of youth suicide have been dramatically increasing, a phenomenon that raises many questions and great concern about preventing this tragic loss of young people in our society. An important means of developing effective prevention strategies is to understand the life course of individuals who are at risk for suicide or nonfatal suicidal behavior. Longitudinal studies, especially those with a prospective research design, are among the most revealing types of investigations to identify risk factors for suicidal behavior. However, some drawbacks in conducting these studies are the labor-intensive efforts needed in maintaining the original sample for follow-up assessments. Changes in life circumstances involving mobility, change of jobs, development of psychiatric problems, stressful life events, and attitudes toward research may be salient factors that decrease subjects' rate of participation. Nevertheless, prospective follow-up studies are invaluable in understanding causal links to suicide and nonfatal suicidal behavior.

This chapter will review information offered from longitudinal studies of children and adolescents who are at risk for suicidal behavior. It will describe the course of suicidal children and adolescents, factors associated with suicidal behavior, and the relation of treatment to youth suicidal behavior.

▼ Past Studies of Outcome

Until the early 1990s, there were relatively few prospective studies of suicidal children or adolescents. These studies had a number of methodological limitations, including small sample sizes, lack of standardized assessment methods, uncontrolled samples, and varied length of follow-up periods. From a historical perspective, these studies alerted the scientific and lay community to the significant morbidity and mortality associated with early-onset suicidal behavior.

Two studies are notable in following up on prepubertal suicidal children. An 18-month follow-up study (Cohen-Sandler et al. 1982) suggested that 20% of suicidal child psychiatric inpatients will demonstrate suicidal acts within less than 2 years. A 2-year follow-up study of a community sample of children (Pfeffer et al. 1988a) reported that 19% of the 67 prepubertal students exhibited suicidal ideation or attempts at follow-up compared with 12% who reported suicidal ideation or behavior at the initial assessment. This study suggested that suicidal tendencies were stable within a 2-year time frame of assessing healthy children in the community. None of the children in these studies committed suicide, although one child in the 18 months follow-up of child psychiatric inpatients died in a boating accident. Stressful life events, treatment utilization, social adjustment, and out-of-home placement were similar during follow-up of the suicidal and nonsuicidal prepubertal psychiatric inpatients (Cohen-Sandler et al. 1982).

Short-term studies of adolescents who attempted suicide reported varied rates of future suicidal acts within 1 year of follow-up. These rates ranged from 14% of 50 adolescents admitted to a general hospital because of a suicide attempt (Hawton et al. 1982) to 42% of 50 adolescent psychiatric inpatients admitted after an acute suicide attempt (Barter et al. 1968). No suicides occurred in these studies. At follow-up, psychiatric patients admitted for a suicide attempt, compared with those admitted for other psychiatric problems, were more frequently not living at home, had a poorer social life, and had more social agency involvements.

Among the intermediate follow-up studies with average follow-ups of 4–7 years, the rate of suicide was low. Suicide occurred in 0.9% of 1,331 adolescent psychiatric inpatients (Kuperman et al. 1988). Four percent of 130 adolescent psychiatric inpatients who attempted suicide committed suicide during follow-up (Nardini-Maillard and Ladame 1980). The highest suicide rate in follow-up was reported for a sample of 122 male adolescent psychiatric inpatients who were hospitalized after a suicide attempt (Motto 1984). Nine percent of these adolescents were identified as having committed suicide using a record linkage methodology for coroner records. Suicide attempt rates during follow-up are not reported in these studies.

Long-term studies involving average follow-up periods of 9–12 years reported suicide rates ranging from 0 to 4.3% (Angle et al. 1983; Otto 1972; Paerregaard 1975). A report of 47 adolescent psychiatric inpatients who attempted suicide noted that 47% experienced a repeat suicide attempt during the follow-up period (Angle et al. 1983).

▼ Past Studies of the Relation of Intervention to Outcome

Data about naturalistic or controlled trials of treatment regarding suicidal behavior in children and adolescents are relatively nonexistent. This is an important area in which investigation needs to be fostered.

Empirically gathered data suggest that preadolescents and adolescents who are psychiatric patients, especially those who have been psychiatrically hospitalized, have higher rates of suicide and suicide attempts than children and adolescents who are not psychiatric patients. For example, Kuperman et al. (1988) reported a nine times greater rate of suicide among former child and adolescent psychiatric inpatients than among youth in the general population.

This finding probably reflects the higher degree of risk associated with the psychosocial and psychopathological histories of psychiatrically hospitalized children and adolescents rather than adverse effects of psychiatric hospitalization. This is further illustrated by 8- to 10-year follow-up data on a group of 77 adolescent psychiatric inpatients. At follow-up, one-quarter of the patients diagnosed with bipolar disorder during the index hospitalization committed suicide (Welner et al. 1979). One-tenth of 10 adolescents who had only partial remission of major depressive disorder committed suicide during the follow-up period. This study amplifies on the high risk for suicidal acts that exists in children and adolescents who have mood disorders.

▼ Other Factors Influencing Outcome

Two studies conducted before the 1990s utilized controlled research methodology to identify risk factors, other than a history of suicidal behavior, for future suicidal acts. Pfeffer et al. (1988a) reported on variables that significantly differentiated 13 children who either thought about or attempted suicide at a 2-year follow-up from nonsuicidal children at the time of follow-up. All children were initially selected from the community and had no history of psychiatric evaluation or treatment. Factors that distinguished between children who were suicidal and those who were not suicidal at follow-up were early history of depression and other symptoms of psychopathology within the 2 years preceding the suicidal behavior at follow-up.

This study pointed out that among prepubertal children in the community, symptoms of psychopathology, especially those related to mood disorder, were significant risk factors for future suicidal ideation or acts within a 2-year period of follow-up. This study also highlighted the persistence of psychiatric symptomatology, which enhanced risk for suicidal tendencies among those children. For example, of the children who were initially diagnosed with a psychiatric disorder, approximately 70% were given a psychiatric diagnosis at 2-year follow-up. The most frequent disorders present initially and at 2-year follow-up were overanxious, dysthymic, or specific developmental disorder. When children who were persistently non-suicidal in the 2-year course of study were compared with those who reported suicidal ideas or acts at the 2-year follow-up but not initially, factors that were associated with the development of suicidal tendencies in these prepubertal children were presence of assaultive behavior at the initial assessment and symptoms of psychopathology before the follow-up suicidal behavior, especially those of depressive disorders. This study clearly suggests that among relatively healthy children, those vulnerable to future suicidal tendencies exhibit psychiatric symptomatology, specifically involving depressive and aggressive features.

Another notable prospective study conducted before the 1990s involved a sample of 122 male adolescents who were psychiatrically hospitalized after a suicide attempt (Motto 1984). These adolescents were followed up within an average of 7 years by means of record linkage methods using the coroner's records to identify those who committed suicide. Many variables were directly evaluated at the time of these adolescents' psychiatric hospitalization. Those that were identified as being associated with suicide were clear communication of intent to die at the time of the initial suicide attempt, fear of losing one's mind, increased amount of sleep, apathy and psychomotor retardation, feelings of hopelessness, attempts to seek help accompanied by negative attitude toward the caregiver, inability to communicate feelings and thoughts to others, and possession of insufficient financial resources. In general, those adolescents who committed suicide had early features of physiological problems, ability to communicate suicidal intent, help-seeking behavior, hopelessness, and intense fears about their mental stability. These findings suggest extensive psychological vulnerability among adolescents who commit suicide.

Little data exist from prospective studies conducted before 1990 that identify stressful events as risk factors for youth suicidal behavior. A unique report (Salk et al. 1985) described prenatal and neonatal factors predictive of youth suicide. Forty-six factors involving prenatal, birth, and neonatal events of 52 adolescents who committed suicide were compared with such factors in a demographically matched sample of nonsuicidal adolescents. The adolescents who committed suicide had significantly more adverse prenatal, birth, and neonatal factors than those who were not suicidal. The most common early risk factors for suicide were infant respiratory distress for more than 1 hour at birth, no maternal antenatal care before 20 weeks of pregnancy, and chronic disease of the mother during the pregnancy. The mechanisms that underlie the associations of these early factors to suicide years later require additional study.

Prospective studies to evaluate the relative risk of family and biological factors for child or adolescent suicidal behavior have not been reported. Information has been derived from cross-sectional and retrospective accounts that identify these factors as correlates of youth suicidal behavior. Studies suggest that suicidal behavior, violence, and abuse in families are related to child and adolescent suicidal behavior (Pfeffer 1989). Furthermore, although deficits in the functioning of serotonin, a neurotransmitter that is widespread in the human brain, have been reported to be associated with suicidal behavior in adults (Mann et al. 1989), no prospective study of children or adolescents has evaluated this for youth suicidal behavior.

This section highlighted the dearth of prospective studies, especially before 1990, that focused on evaluating psychosocial and biological risk factors for youth suicidal behavior. Most studies of child and adolescent suicidal behavior that were conducted before 1990 investigated correlates of youth suicidal behavior by means of cross-sectional and psychological autopsy methodology. As a result, the data gleaned from research studies were primarily retrospective. However, these studies were seminal in elucidating important hypotheses regarding risk factors for youth suicidal behavior, which became the focus of longitudinal studies whose results began to be reported in the early 1990s. These more current studies are discussed in the next section.

▼ Current Prospective Studies

In recent years exciting new prospective studies of children and adolescents who are at risk for suicidal behavior have emerged. These studies utilize improved research methodology involving systematic standard assessments, appropriate statistical analyses for

longitudinal follow-up, and adequately sized comparison populations. The most important aspect of these studies is that many have
their initial phase of evaluation during the prepubertal stage of development. Thus, prospective data have been collected with reliable evidence about the early development of these youngsters. It
is notable that prospective studies have been conducted with children and adolescents who have a range of severity of psychopathology. Some studies focus attention on youth who are psychiatric
patients and who are documented to have serious forms of psychopathology. Other studies utilize community samples of children and
adolescents whose level of psychopathology is relatively low. The
importance of studying youth with varied degrees of psychopathology and social circumstances is that these populations afford the
possibility of validating findings of risk factors for suicidal behavior.
The studies described below are those that are derived from samples of psychiatric patients and others that involve youth selected
from the community.

Psychiatric Patients

A study that is unique in focusing on the prospective follow-up of
prepubertal suicidal children has been reported by Pfeffer et al.
(1991, 1992, 1993). In this study, 133 prepubertal children were
followed prospectively for an average of over 7 years. Initially, the
prepubertal children were grouped as 25 psychiatric inpatients who
had attempted suicide, 28 psychiatric inpatients who reported suicidal ideation, 16 nonsuicidal psychiatric inpatients, and 64 children selected from the community to match the demographic
characteristics of the psychiatric inpatients. A number of important
results were derived from this study.

First, history of suicidal ideation or a suicide attempt during
prepuberty is a strong risk factor for a suicide attempt in adolescence. Specifically, prepubertal psychiatric inpatients who
attempted suicide were found to be at over 6 times greater risk than
the prepubertal community sample for a suicide attempt in adolescence. In addition, prepubertal psychiatric inpatients who reported
a suicidal ideation, compared with the children selected from the

community, were at greater than 3.6 times risk for a future suicide attempt. This study identified the predictive validity of suicidal ideation or a suicide attempt in prepuberty for suicidal acts in adolescence.

Second, presence of a mood disorder, substance abuse disorder, stressful life events, and poor social adjustment are other risk factors for a suicide attempt in adolescence. Specifically, the strongest risk factors for a suicide attempt in adolescence are poor social adjustment and presence of a mood disorder, especially when both factors are present shortly before a suicide attempt. This study pointed out that factors proximal to a suicide attempt are stronger risk factors than those distal to a suicide attempt. An important clinical implication involves the need to assess current psychosocial and psychopathological status in evaluations of youth suicidal risk.

Third, this naturalistic study suggested that both suicidal and nonsuicidal psychiatric inpatients had longer psychiatric treatment histories over their youthful lifetimes. In fact, some of the youngsters who attempted suicide carried out their suicidal acts while in intensive treatment. This study highlighted the need for controlled treatment trials of suicidal behavior in children and adolescents.

Prospective follow-up studies of adolescent and young adult psychiatric inpatients who exhibit suicidal tendencies are relatively few. An important case-control prospective study to determine factors associated with suicide in 15- to 24-year-old patients who attempted suicide was conducted in England (Hawton et al. 1993). This study resembles the research design of the record linkage study of male adolescent psychiatric inpatients who attempted suicide that was conducted by Motto (1984). In this English study, 62 youths admitted between 1968 and 1985 to a regional poisoning treatment center because of deliberate self-poisoning or self-injury committed suicide. These youths were compared with 124 patients of similar age who did not die.

Several factors identified during index treatment were identified as being associated with subsequent suicide. Low socioeconomic status increased risk for suicide by threefold. Unemployment imparted an almost three times greater risk for suicide. Previous psychiatric inpatient treatment increased risk for suicide by approximately five times. Substance abuse increased risk for suicide by over three times, whereas personality disorder increased risk two times. A history of a previous suicide attempt increased risk for suicide by over two times. However, the strongest predictors of suicide were identified to be substance abuse, which raised risk almost fourfold, and a history of psychiatric hospitalization, which elevated risk almost four times. An important implication of this study for suicide prevention is that communication between professionals who treat youths who attempt suicide and professionals who treat youthful substance abusers will enhance the likelihood of identifying and appropriately treating youth who are most at risk for suicide.

Brent et al. (1993a) highlighted some important issues regarding the high risk of suicidal adolescents for repeat suicidal acts. In this study of 48 adolescents who were psychiatrically hospitalized after a suicide attempt, 33 adolescent psychiatric inpatients with a recent history of suicidal ideation, and 53 adolescent psychiatric inpatients who were not suicidal, almost 15% of the psychiatric patients made a suicide attempt within 6 months of being discharged from the hospital. Of these 13 adolescents, 12 had been hospitalized for either suicidal ideation or a suicide attempt. Other risk factors for the postdischarge suicide attempt were major depressive disorder at admission, a depressive disorder that persisted after hospitalization, mood disorder that was comorbid with other disorders, family stress such as death of a relative, or financial problems. It was noteworthy that those adolescents who attempted suicide at follow-up were more likely to have been treated with antidepressants. Another treatment issue suggested by this study was the lower rate of family therapy for those adolescents who attempted suicide after hospitalization.

These three studies of suicidal children and suicidal adolescents point out the high risk for future suicidal behavior imparted to these youngsters. These studies emphasize the important role of a mood disorder in enhancing suicidal risk.

Other prospective studies (Harrington et al. 1990; Kovacs et al. 1993; Rao et al. 1993) support the importance of prepubertal major depressive disorder as a risk factor for suicide attempts in adolescence and suicide in late adolescence and young adulthood. For example, Kovacs et al. (1993) reported that although the rate of suicide attempts was 9% among prepubertal psychiatric outpatients with depressive and nondepressive disorders, the rate increased to 24% by late adolescence. Major depressive disorder and dysthymic disorder increased risk for a future suicide attempt. Furthermore, similar to the report by Brent et al. (1993a), Kovacs et al. (1993) reported an increased risk for a suicide attempt in adolescence when a mood disorder was comorbid with conduct and/or substance abuse disorders.

Myers et al. (1991) conducted a yearly follow-up for 3 years of 76 children and adolescents who were initially diagnosed with major depressive disorder. Similar to the findings of Kovacs et al. (1993), Myers et al. (1991) reported that 72% reported suicidal ideation or suicidal acts during the 3-year course of study. This high rate of suicidal tendencies among depressed children and adolescents validates other results relating suicidal behavior to depressive symptomatology. Myers et al. (1991) also noted that the initial rate of 66% for suicidal tendencies dropped to 31% in the first year of follow-up and thereafter remained stable at 28% and 26% for the second and third years of follow-up, respectively. Most of the suicidal tendencies reported in the follow-up assessments were among the youths who were initially suicidal. Children and adolescents who were initially nonsuicidal remained nonsuicidal during follow-up. In general, suicidal behavior tended to remit and recur. Also, there appeared to be a decreasing strength of influence of initial suicidal status on later suicidal status. Other factors that predicted suicidal status in follow-up were severity of initial suicidal state and presence of anger initially.

Emphasis on the significance of major depressive disorder was highlighted also in the results of a follow-up in late adolescence and young adulthood (Rao et al. 1993). This study identified that the seven suicidal youth deaths were all among late adolescents and young adults who had a major depressive disorder as children (Rao et al. 1993). Most of these suicide victims had recurrent depressive symptoms and had a mood disorder at the time of their suicide.

Relatively little has been reported about features of treatment of suicidal youth. Trautman et al. (1993) compared the attendance at psychiatric outpatient treatment sessions for 115 consecutively admitted 10- to 18-year-old minority youth who had attempted suicide and 110 age-matched minority psychiatric outpatients who were nonsuicidal. The youths were predominantly Hispanic and female. Although the subjects who had attempted suicide and those who had not both had high drop-out rates for treatment, those who had attempted suicide dropped out significantly earlier and kept fewer treatment appointments. These results are similar to those reported by Pfeffer et al. (1988b), suggesting that adolescent psychiatric inpatients who attempt suicide, compared with nonsuicidal adolescent inpatients, sign themselves out of the hospital more frequently and earlier.

Community Samples

From a public health perspective in which primary prevention of suicidal behavior is an important goal, investigation of children in the general community for risk of suicidal behavior is a first step in conceptualizing and implementing suicide prevention programs. This section will discuss longitudinal studies that provide insights about vulnerability factors to suicidal behavior identified among children and adolescents in the general community. These populations are predominantly nonreferred samples for psychiatric care.

Suicidal ideation, rather than suicidal acts, is the predominant suicidal symptom in youth selected from the general community. For example, Garrison et al. (1991) reported that less than 5.5% of 1,073 seventh-grade or eighth-grade students, who were predominantly 12–14 years old, reported serious suicidal ideation each year of a 3-year prospective study. These students were primarily females. In fact, individual students' suicidal status fluctuated rather than being persistent during this 3-year study. The strongest predictor of a particular year's suicidal level was the previous year's severity of depressive symptoms. This finding for suicidal ideation is consistent with the significant association of depressive symptoms and suicidal acts reported for child and adolescent psychiatric patients.

Other samples of youth selected from the general community may be at particular risk for suicidal behavior. For example, Brent et al. (1993b) hypothesized that adolescent friends and acquaintances of adolescents who committed suicide may be at significant risk for suicide attempts or suicide. Seven months after the suicidal death of an adolescent, 146 adolescent friends and acquaintances were evaluated and compared with 146 adolescents who were not exposed to an adolescent who committed suicide. Compared with the nonexposed adolescents, adolescents who were friendly with or were acquainted with an adolescent who committed suicide had significantly more psychiatric symptoms that began after the death. These included symptoms of major depressive disorder, posttraumatic stress disorder, and suicidal ideation with a plan. There was no excessive rate of suicide attempts among the friends or acquaintances of an adolescent suicide victim. No onset of suicidal ideation after the suicide of a friend or acquaintance was associated with the new onset of depressive symptomatology. Although this is a cross-sectional study, follow-up is planned.

A number of issues are raised by this study, especially with respect to the risk for suicidal acts among friends and acquaintances of adolescent suicide victims. A limitation of this study was that only 67% of friends or acquaintances of all suicide victims were evaluated. Therefore, it is possible that those who did not participate may have a different profile of risk for suicidal acts. Given the long duration of depressive symptoms among friends and acquaintances of youth suicide victims, intervention for these depressed adolescents should be offered on an intensive basis to ameliorate mood disorder symptoms and future risk for suicidal behavior. Further follow-up of these adolescents is needed to determine if long-term risk for suicidal acts exists.

Because symptoms of depression are significantly associated with youth suicidal behavior, another community sample that may be at high risk for suicidal behavior are the children of parents with major depressive disorder. Such children, who are at risk for mood and other psychiatric disorders, may report high rates of suicidal tendencies. Weissman et al. (1992) aimed to evaluate whether the offspring of parents with major depressive disorder, compared with offspring of parents without psychopathology, will report higher rates of suicidal behavior. This 2-year prospective study evaluated 174 offspring, ages 6–23 years. During a 2-year follow-up period, all new episodes of suicide attempts, major depression, and anxiety disorders occurred only among the offspring of parents with a history of major depressive disorder. Within the 2 years of follow-up, the suicide attempt rate was 7.8% for offspring of parents with major depressive disorder compared with 1.4% for offspring of parents who were not depressed. Important implications for primary prevention of suicidal behavior is to identify children and adolescents who have parents with a history of major depressive disorder and to follow these youngsters closely in order to identify early risk for suicidal acts. In a similar way, it is important to determine whether other aspects of familial psychopathology enhance risk of offspring for youth suicidal behavior.

Prevention Programs

Since the early 1980s, when the community at large became aware of the national public health problem of youth suicide and nonfatal suicidal behavior, attempts have been undertaken to prevent youth suicide by means of school-based suicide prevention programs. Such programs, developed in schools throughout the United States, have diverse curricula. Most programs have not been evaluated for their efficacy.

Vieland et al. (1991) reported a prospective evaluation of a school-based suicide prevention program for high-school students. The results of the 18-month prospective follow-up assessment suggested that there was no beneficial effect in reducing suicidal morbidity or enhancing help-seeking behavior from a school-based suicide prevention program advertised 18 months before. Adolescents who received the suicide prevention curriculum did not differ from adolescents who attended other schools in which the suicide prevention program was not advertised. The advantage of the relatively long follow-up period in this study was that enough time elapsed to identify a sufficient number of adolescents with suicidal behavior and to compare these rates among adolescents who received and those who did not receive the school-based suicide prevention programs. This study noted that 2.5% of adolescents exposed to this suicide prevention program and 2.7% of adolescents not exposed to the program reported at least one suicide attempt during the 18-month follow-up period.

▼ Summary

There has been a recent burgeoning of prospective studies of children and adolescents at risk for suicidal behavior. This is most probably related to the enhanced knowledge about youth suicidal behavior gleaned from cross-sectional and psychological autopsy studies, which depend heavily on retrospective data. The advantage of prospective studies is in the ability to identify causal links in the evolution of youth suicidal behavior. Since the 1990s, several prospective reports have appeared related to risk for youth suicidal behavior. For example, Table 6–1 highlights the few recent systematic follow-up reports of suicidal youth.

Important results of recent studies are that a history of psychiatric hospitalization, presence of mood disorders, and substance abuse are significant risk factors for youth suicidal behavior. Furthermore, history of suicidal behavior is a consistent risk factor for repeated suicide attempts or suicide.

Information about the efficacy of treatment is lacking. The naturalistic design of most of these studies has been valuable in documenting the types of treatments received by children and adolescents who report suicidal ideation or attempts. However, only prospective controlled treatment studies will be able to clarify types of treatments that are most effective to reduce risk for youth suicidal behavior. Such studies are urgently needed.

Finally, it is hoped by everyone that youth suicidal behavior is preventable. Prospective studies can be helpful in identifying which processes at specific stages of development require most preventive intervention in order to reduce suicidal risk. Prospective approaches should be a major component of all suicide prevention programs.

Table 6-1. Recent prospective studies of suicidal youth

Author (year)	Number of subjects	Sample	Follow-up duration (years)	Risk factors for suicidal behavior
Pfeffer et al. 1991, 1992, 1993	133	25 prepubertal suicide attempter inpatients 28 prepubertal suicide ideator inpatients 16 nonsuicidal patients 64 nonpatients	6–8	Suicidal ideation, suicide attempt, mood disorder, substance abuse, poor social adjustment, stressful life events
Hawton et al. 1993	186	62 adolescent suicide victims 124 adolescent suicide attempter patients	17	Suicide attempt, susbstance abuse, psychiatric hospitalization, unemployment, low socio-economic status
Brent et al. 1993a	134	48 adolescent suicide attempter inpatients 33 adolescent suicide ideator inpatients 53 adolescent nonsuicidal inpatients	0.5	Suicidal ideation, suicide attempt, mood disorder, family stress

▼ References

Angle CR, O'Brien TP, McIntire MS: Adolescent self-poisoning: a nine-year follow-up. J Dev Behav Pediatr 4:83–87, 1983

Barter JT, Swaback DO, Todd D: Adolescent suicide attempts: a follow-up study of hospitalized patients. Arch Gen Psychiatry 19:523–527, 1968

Brent DA, Kolko DJ, Wartella ME, et al: Adolescent psychiatric inpatients' risk of suicide attempt at 6 month follow-up. J Am Acad Child Adolesc Psychiatry 32:95–105, 1993a

Brent DA, Perper JA, Moritz G, et al: Psychiatric sequelae to loss of an adolescent peer to suicide. J Am Acad Child Adolesc Psychiatry 32:509–517, 1993b

Cohen-Sandler R, Berman AL, King RA: A follow-up study of hospitalized suicidal children. J Am Acad Child Psychiatry 21:398–403, 1982

Garrison CZ, Addy CL, Jackson KL, et al: A longitudinal study of suicidal ideation in young adolescents. J Am Acad Child Adolesc Psychiatry 30:597–603, 1991

Harrington R, Fudge H, Rutter M, et al: Adult outcomes of childhood and adolescent depression. Arch Gen Psychiatry 47:465–473, 1990

Hawton K, Osborn M, O'Grady J, et al: Classification of adolescents who take overdoses. Br J Psychiatry 140:124–131, 1982

Hawton K, Fagg J, Platt S, et al: Factors associated with suicide after parasuicide in young people. BMJ 306:1641–1644, 1993

Kovacs M, Goldston D, Gatsonis C: Suicidal behaviors and childhood onset depressive disorders: a longitudinal investigation. J Am Acad Child Adolesc Psychiatry 32:8–20, 1993

Kuperman S, Black DW, Burns TL: Excess mortality among formerly hospitalized child psychiatric patients. Arch Gen Psychiatry 45:277–282, 1988

Mann JJ, DeMeo MD, Keilp JG, et al: Biological correlates of suicidal behavior in youth, in Suicide Among Youth: Perspectives On Risk and Prevention. Edited by Pfeffer CR. Washington, DC, American Psychiatric Press Inc., 1989, pp 185–202

Motto JA: Suicide in male adolescents, in Suicide in the Young. Edited by Sudak HS, Ford AB, Rushforth NB. Boston, MA, J Wright-PSG, Inc., 1984, pp 227–244

Myers K, McCauley E, Calderon R, et al: The 3-year longitudinal course of suicidality and predictive factors for subsequent suicidality in youths with major depressive disorder. J Am Acad Child Adolesc Psychiatry 30:804–810, 1991

Nardini-Maillard D, Ladame FG: The results of a follow-up study of suicidal adolescents. J Adolesc 3:253–260, 1980

Otto U: Suicidal acts by children and adolescents: a follow-up study. Acta Psychiatr Scand Suppl 233:7–123, 1972

Paerregaard G: Suicide among attempted suicides: a two year follow-up. Suicide 5:140–144, 1975

Pfeffer CR: Life stress and family risk factors for youth fatal and nonfatal suicidal behavior, in Suicide Among Youth: Perspectives on Risk and Prevention. Edited by Pfeffer CR. Washington, DC, American Psychiatric Press Inc., 1989, pp 143–164

Pfeffer CR, Lipkins R, Plutchik R, et al: Normal children at risk for suicidal behavior: a two-year follow-up study. J Am Acad Child Adolesc Psychiatry 27:34–41, 1988a

Pfeffer CR, Newcorn J, Kaplan G, et al: Suicidal behavior in adolescent psychiatric inpatients. J Am Acad Child Adolesc Psychiatry 27:357–361, 1988b

Pfeffer CR, Klerman GL, Hurt SW, et al: Suicidal children grow up: demographic and clinical risk factors for adolescent suicide attempts. J Am Acad Child Adolesc Psychiatry 30:609–616, 1991

Pfeffer CR, Peskin JR, Siefker CA: Suicidal children grow up: treatment during follow-up. J Am Acad Child Adolesc Psychiatry 31:679–685, 1992

Pfeffer CR, Klerman GL, Hurt SW, et al: Suicidal children grow up: rates and psychosocial risk factors for suicide attempts during follow-up. J Am Acad Child Adolesc Psychiatry 32:106–113, 1993

Rao U, Weissman MM, Martin JA, et al: Childhood depression and risk of suicide: a preliminary report of a longitudinal study. J Am Acad Child Adolesc Psychiatry 32:21–27, 1993

Salk L, Lipsitt LP, Sturner WQ, et al: Relationship to maternal and perinatal conditions to eventual adolescent suicide. Lancet 1:624–627, 1985

Trautman PD, Stewart N, Morishima A: Are adolescent suicide attempters noncompliant with outpatient care? J Am Acad Child Adolesc Psychiatry 32:89–94, 1993

Vieland V, Whittle B, Garland A, et al: The impact of curriculum-based suicide prevention programs for teenagers: an 18-month follow-up. J Am Acad Child Adolesc Psychiatry 30:811–815, 1991

Weissman MM, Fendrich M, Warner V, et al: Incidence of psychiatric disorder in offspring at high and low risk for depression. J Am Acad Child Adolesc Psychiatry 31:640–648, 1992

Welner A, Welner Z, Fishman R: Psychiatric adolescent inpatients: eight to ten year follow-up. Arch Gen Psychiatry 36:698–700, 1979

Chapter 7

Childhood Anxiety Disorders

**Diane Majcher, M.D., M.S., and
Mark H. Pollack, M.D.**

Anxiety disorders are among the most common psychiatric disorders of childhood and adolescence (Anderson et al. 1987; Keller et al. 1992; McGee et al. 1990). Kashani and Orvaschel (1988) reported that 17.3% of a sample of 14- to 16-year-olds met criteria for one or more anxiety disorders, with 8.7% experiencing significant impairment. A study by Keller et al. (1992) found that 14% of children ages 6–19 had a lifetime history of anxiety disorders. Anxiety disorders occur twice as frequently as attention deficit disorder in children (Popper 1993).

Anxious children are more likely than nonanxious children to show disturbance of mood, conduct, and social functioning and may be at increased risk for adjustment problems in adulthood (Coolidge et al. 1964; Strauss et al. 1988; Waldron 1976). Anxiety disorders in childhood are often chronic and recurrent and may cause long-term impairment in functioning, including persistent academic and vocational underachievement, increased medical care utilization, and interference with the acquisition of appropriate developmental skills, such as social skills (Kane and Kendall 1989; Keller et al. 1992; Popper 1993).

Adult patients with panic disorder and agoraphobia who have a history of childhood anxiety disorders have a more chronic course of illness, and are at increased risk for comorbid anxiety and for affective and personality dysfunction (Pollack et al. 1990, 1992). Panic disorder with onset in childhood or adolescence is associated with suicidal thoughts and suicide attempts (Weissman et al. 1989). Markowitz et al. (1989) note that 29% of people with panic disorder use emergency departments for the treatment of emotional problems, as compared with 12% with major depression or other psychiatric disorders and 3% of those with no psychiatric disorder. It is important to identify children at risk for developing anxiety disorders in order to reduce distress during childhood, facilitate appropriate development during childhood, and, potentially, to prevent complications during adulthood.

▼ Difficulties in Studying Childhood Anxiety Disorders

There has been a relative paucity of studies examining anxiety disorders in children and adolescents, and fewer looking at the long-term outcome of these disorders. Much of the existing research has methodological problems such as small sample size, wide developmental age range of subjects, use of either child or parent alone as informant, and lack of controls and standardized diagnostic and assessment instruments. Many of the large epidemiological studies occurred before the use of the standardized diagnostic categories identified in DSM-III (American Psychiatric Association 1980) and report estimates of global maladjustment rather than prevalence of specific disorders (Abe and Masui 1981; Agras et al. 1969; Earls 1980; Kastrup 1976; Lapouse and Monk 1958; Richman et al. 1975; Werry and Quay 1971). Continued refinement in diagnostic criteria may limit the applicability of prior studies on course of illness and treatment response.

Syndromes that have been the subject of more extensive study, such as school refusal, actually reflect a heterogeneous group of disorders including separation anxiety disorder (SAD), major depression, and conduct disorder rather than a single diagnostic category (Popper 1993). Many earlier studies have used the terms *separation anxiety disorder, school refusal,* or *school phobia* interchangeably when actually about 27% of children with SAD do not present with school reluctance or refusal (Last et al. 1987b). Such diagnostic heterogeneity hinders interpretation of data on treatment response and long-term outcome.

Understanding of the long-term course of childhood pathology is hindered by the current lack of clarity regarding the equivalence and temporal continuity of childhood and adult diagnoses. Bernstein and Borchardt (1991) observed that the separation of the anxiety disorders in DSM-III-R (American Psychiatric Association 1987) into disorders of childhood and adolescence and disorders of adulthood facilitated research on anxiety in children by removing the constraints of adult criteria. However, promoting a separate focus on the childhood disorders may hinder our understanding of the longitudinal course of anxiety disorders. The confusion over the continuity of anxiety disorders is exemplified by the relationship between overanxious disorder (OAD) in childhood and adult generalized anxiety disorder (GAD). The DSM-III-R criteria for GAD specify that at least two life events are unrealistic and excessive sources of worry, whereas criteria for childhood OAD require that the worry about future events be more global, thus concentrating on potentially independent foci of anxiety, which may not identify the same individuals. In addition, only 20% of adults with GAD in one study reported childhood or adolescent onset of symptoms, suggesting that OAD is not a necessary or specific antecedent for adult GAD (Thyer et al. 1985).

The issue of developmental age-appropriate behavior also presents several problems for research on outcome of childhood anxiety difficulties. Developmentally appropriate anxiety symptoms in young children (e.g., fear of the dark and stranger anxiety) may be misdiagnosed as evidence of an anxiety disorder. Also, children may present with different symptom constellations when distressed than adults, contributing to diagnostic confusion. For example, young children with posttraumatic stress disorder (PTSD) may relive the past through the action of repetitive play rather than through flashbacks and may tend to focus on somatic complaints rather than the symptoms of increased arousal noted in adults (American Psychiatric Association 1987). Some investigators believe panic attacks to be rare before puberty (D. F. Klein et al. 1992) and have posited separation anxiety as a phobic manifestation of panic disorder in childhood (Abelson and Alessi 1992). Some young children may not have the cognitive capacity to describe spontaneous physical symptoms or acknowledge fears of losing control or going crazy, as is necessary to meet the diagnostic criteria of panic attacks in adulthood (Nelles and Barlow 1988). Although anxious children exhibit physiological responses, such as elevated heart rates, which distinguish them from nonanxious children (Beidel 1988), they may not report more physical symptoms than nonanxious children (Laurent et al. 1993).

There may be certain at-risk periods for the development of pathological anxiety during the life cycle, corresponding to changes in neurophysiological and other developmental factors. Charney et al. (1990) proposed a developmental theory of panic disorder in which alterations in noradrenergic function over time may account for the onset and decline of panic symptoms. Locus coeruleus (LC) neuronal activity in young animals is low until maturity, when greater LC activity is observed (Kimura and Nakamura 1985, 1987; Williams and Marshall 1987). The number and activity of LC neurons decreases with aging, correlating with diminished noradrenergic activity (Bondareff and Mountjoy 1986; Feldman et al. 1984; Olpe and Steinmann 1982; Robinson et al. 1972). The typical onset of panic attacks in adolescence or early adulthood may correspond with maturation of the LC-noradrenergic system; immature or diminished LC activity may account for why onset of panic appears rarely in the very young or elderly and is consistent with assertions that phobic anxiety and temperamental inhibition may be more common in children than frank panic attacks. In addition, animal studies suggest that adverse experience during infancy may have long-term effects on central noradrenergic and serotoninergic systems and may determine subsequent susceptibility to anxiety and affective disorders and pharmacological responsivity (Rosenblum et al. 1994).

Comorbid anxiety disorders (Kashani and Orvaschel 1988; Last et al. 1987a), depression (Bernstein and Borchardt 1991), attention deficit disorder (Munir et al. 1987), and behavioral disorders (Last et al. 1992) are common in anxious children and adolescents and contribute to the difficulty in studying the long-term outcome of the anxiety disorders. Last et al. (1987a) reported that one-third of outpatient children with a primary diagnosis of SAD had a concurrent diagnosis of OAD, one-third of primary OAD patients were comorbid for social phobia, and one-quarter were comorbid for avoidant disorder. This overlap complicates the attempt to study the course and outcome of specific anxiety disorders. In addition, findings from clinic samples representing more complex populations (Berkson 1946) may not reflect the naturalistic course and outcome of anxiety disorders in the general population.

▼ The Relationship Between Childhood and Adult AnxietyDisorders

Ideally, the best way to understand the relationship between childhood and adult anxiety disorders is through the use of long-term prospective studies. There has been a relative paucity of prospective follow-up of afflicted children utilizing current diagnostic categories for childhood anxiety disorders; retrospective reclassification of subjects from pre–DSM-III epidemiological studies may be subject to significant error. Most of our current knowledge on the relationship between childhood and adult anxiety disorders is based on information from studies using retrospective reports of childhood from adults with anxiety disorders, family studies of afflicted adults and children, and a small number of short-term prospective studies. The following sections will review studies examining the long-term outcome of childhood anxiety disorders, including separation anxiety disorder, overanxious disorder, avoidant disorder, panic disorder, agoraphobia, social phobia, simple phobia, and PTSD.

Retrospective Studies of Childhood History

Adults with panic disorder often report the onset of anxiety difficulties in childhood or adolescence. In the Epidemiologic Catchment Area study (von Korff et al. 1985), 18% of adults with panic
disorder reported experiencing panic attacks before age 10, and 7%
reported experiencing panic attacks between the ages of 10 and 15.
Breier et al. (1984) found in their study of 60 adults with agoraphobia, mixed phobia, and/or panic disorder that 28% experienced
their first panic attack before age 20. Through a retrospective chart
review of 62 subjects, Thyer et al. (1985) found that 38% of the
adults with panic disorder experienced their first panic attack before age 20 and 11% experienced before the age of 10.

In one of the earliest studies on the onset of adult anxiety disorders, Klein (1964) observed that 50% of a sample of adult panic
disorder patients with agoraphobia or anticipatory anxiety reported
symptoms of separation anxiety and difficulty adjusting to school
as children. These subjects continued to have symptoms of separation anxiety throughout their lives and experienced panic attacks
under conditions of separation and bereavement. In another study,
Gittelman-Klein and Klein (1973) noted that 50% of adult panic
disorder patients had histories of SAD, fearfulness, dependency,
school adjustment difficulties, and phobia during childhood. In a
prospective study, Rutter and Sandberg (1985) suggest an association between juvenile-onset separation anxiety and adult panic disorder or agoraphobia. Perugi et al. (1988) and Ayuso et al. (1989)
reported that panic disorder and phobic avoidance occurred at an
earlier age in adults with a history of childhood separation anxiety
or school phobia. Rosenbaum et al. (1993) found that 75% of children with separation anxiety at 21 months of age had agoraphobia
at 7.5 years of age, whereas only 7% of children without separation
anxiety at baseline were observed to have developed agoraphobia at
follow-up.

However, early suggestions (Klein 1964) positing a specific link
between separation anxiety in childhood and adult panic disorder
have been broadened to include a more general link between pathological anxiety during childhood and adulthood. Aronson and Logue
(1987) reported elevated rates of anxiety disorders in a retro-

spective assessment of panic disorder patients, with the incidence of OAD (9%) close to twice that of SAD. Berg et al. (1974b), comparing 786 agoraphobic females with 58 nonagoraphobic female psychiatric outpatients, and Tyrer and Tyrer (1974), comparing 60 phobic, 60 anxious, and 120 depressed adult patients, found a history of school phobia equally common in all groups, although the latter investigators did note a nonsignificant tendency for more childhood school refusal in phobic patients. Both groups of investigators concluded that there was a nonspecific link between childhood school refusal and adult neurotic illness. Berg (1976) also observed that agoraphobic women with a childhood history of school phobia had an earlier age at onset of agoraphobia, more severe symptoms, and bore more school-phobic children than those without school phobia.

Raskin et al. (1982) found no differences between patients with panic disorder or GAD in terms of a childhood history of early SAD, long-term separation before age 10, or separation causing exacerbation of symptoms, providing further support for a more nonspecific link between separation anxiety and later psychiatric illness. For panic disorder patients, childhood anxiety difficulties may be particularly associated with agoraphobia (Klein 1984). Deltito et al. (1986) noted that 60% of patients with panic disorder and agoraphobia had histories of school refusal compared with none of those with panic alone.

In an ongoing study of adult panic disorder patients, Pollack et al. (1990, 1992) reported that a history of any childhood anxiety disorder—including SAD, OAD, social phobia, or avoidant disorder—was associated with increased rates of comorbid adult anxiety disorders and apparent Axis II pathology. All of these factors were associated with a more chronic course of panic disorder in adulthood. Sixty-eight percent of patients with a comorbid anxiety disorder had a history of childhood anxiety. For many of these patients, the childhood anxiety disorders apparently remained unsuccessfully treated: 61% of patients with childhood social phobia were socially phobic as adults. OAD in childhood was associated with elevated rates of GAD (35%) and social phobia (58%) in adult patients. Patients with childhood anxiety had greater agoraphobic avoidance as adults, suggesting that early anxiety experiences may contribute to patterns of avoidance maintained through adulthood. Hypotheses regarding early learned patterns of avoidance in response to anxiety are also consistent with findings of higher levels of anxiety sensitivity in patients with a childhood history of anxiety disorders (Otto et al. 1994). Anxiety sensitivity is a fear of anxiety symptoms or a tendency to respond anxiously to sensations of arousal (Reiss et al. 1986). Patients with significant childhood anxiety may have developed anxiety sensitivity during childhood as a result of their repeated negative anxiety experiences or may have become more anxiety sensitive over time. Anxiety sensitivity may be one mediating factor in the development or maintenance of panic disorder in patients with childhood anxiety difficulties.

▼ Family Studies

The presumption that many of the anxiety disorders are familial and probably have a genetic basis has been reinforced through family and twin studies of panic disorder (Crowe et al. 1983; Torgerson 1983). Family studies that evaluate the prevalence of anxiety disorders in the children of adult patients with anxiety disorders ("top down") and the parents of children with anxiety disorders ("bottom up") are also consistent with a relationship between childhood and adult illness, although the specific nature of the familial transmission (i.e., for a specific disorder or a general predisposition for pathological anxiety) is an area of ongoing investigation.

Top-Down Studies

Berg (1976) found a 14% prevalence of school phobia in the 11- to 15-year-old children of a large sample of agoraphobic women, a rate higher than expected in the general population. In a later study, Weissman et al. (1984) noted that the rate of anxiety symptoms was much higher among the children of depressed parents with a history of panic disorder or agoraphobia than among the children of pure depressive individuals or control subjects. However, in a smaller study, Turner et al. (1987) found an increased risk of anxiety disorders in the children of parents with both anxiety disorders and dysthymia, leaving open the question of whether parental affective disorder is also associated with increased risk of anxiety disorders in the offspring. Different adult anxiety disorders may be variably associated with anxiety in the offspring. For example, in one study, the offspring of parents with panic disorder but not GAD were at significantly greater risk for separation anxiety (Weissman et al. 1984).

Bottom-Up Studies

Gittelman-Klein (1975) observed that separation anxiety was more frequent in the parents of school-phobic children than in the parents of hyperactive children (19% vs. 2%). Although Berg et al. (1974a) did not find a significant difference in the prevalence of psychiatric illness in mothers of hospitalized adolescents with school phobias compared with those who had other problems, potential differences may have been obscured by the failure to exclude patients with anxiety symptoms from the comparison group. More recently, Last et al. (1987c) compared parents of children who had SAD and/or OAD with parents of children who had behavior disorders and found an increased lifetime prevalence of anxiety disorders in the mothers of the children with anxiety disorders. Last and Strauss (1990) found an elevated rate (33%) of panic disorder in the mothers but not in the fathers of children with panic disorder, compared with rates observed for mothers of children with other anxiety disorders (10.9%), mothers of children with attention-deficit/hyperactivity disorder (ADHD) (2.5%), and mothers of healthy children (1.9%). Last et al. (1987c) also reported that 83% of the mothers of children with SAD and/or OAD had a lifetime history of an anxiety disorder, with 57% of the mothers presenting with an anxiety disorder at the same time their children were seen for similar problems. Last et al. (1991) observed an increased risk of anxiety disorders in the first- and second-degree male relatives of children with anxiety disorders compared with both ADHD and normal control groups; female relatives did not demonstrate differences from the ADHD group, although rates were increased in the relatives of both patient groups.

▼ Long-Term Outcome

Studies of Anxiety Traits

Several studies suggest that anxiety symptoms in children, including fears and shyness, are relatively stable over time. For instance, in an epidemiological study conducted in the Isle of Wight, Rutter and Sandberg (1985) reported that children who had an "emotional" disorder (i.e., anxiety and/or depression) at age 11 were twice as likely than the rest of the population to have nonconduct emotional disturbances at age 15. However, a questionnaire study and 7-year follow-up of parents of children between ages 2 and 6 (Fischer et al. 1984) suggested that anxiety symptoms in children did not remain stable over time. This latter study may have underestimated pathology by relying on parental report rather than on direct assessment of the children used in the Isle of Wight study.

Behavioral Inhibition and Anxiety Disorders

An animal model for pathological anxiety has been developed by Suomi (1986), who has identified a subgroup of rhesus monkeys who are temperamentally fearful and hyperreactive to stimuli from birth to adulthood and whose progeny demonstrate the same abnormalities. This animal model supports a genetic basis for anxiety-like disorders and the persistence of anxious symptomatology throughout the life span.

In humans, one line of investigation has examined temperament in children, including the offspring of adult anxiety patients, and noted parallels to Suomi's work. Behavioral inhibition (BI) to the unfamiliar is a laboratory-based temperamental construct characterized by the consistent tendency from early in life to display fear and withdrawal in novel or unfamiliar situations (Kagan et al. 1988). Children identified as behaviorally inhibited at age 21 months have been described by their parents as having been irritable, colicky, and sleepless in the first weeks and months of life, suggesting that these children may have been born with a more arousable nervous system (Rosenbaum et al. 1993). Kagan and Snidman (1991) observed that

4-month-olds who displayed a combination of high motor activity and frequent crying in response to such unfamiliar stimulation as toys, mobiles, and vocalizations, were more fearful of unfamiliar events when reevaluated at 9 and 14 months of age. Biederman et al. (1993) also found that the presence of BI at age 21 months was predictive of anxiety disorders 10 years later, thus demonstrating a continuity of psychopathology of increasing severity over time.

Biederman et al. (1993) examined pooled baseline and 3-year follow-up data of the Kagan epidemiological general population cohort sample and an at-risk group, the offspring of parents receiving treatment for panic and agoraphobic disorders. At baseline they noted that inhibited children, compared with noninhibited children, had significantly higher rates of multiple (≥ 2) anxiety disorders. At follow-up, the inhibited group had significantly higher rates of multiple psychiatric disorders (≥ 4), including multiple anxiety disorders (≥ 2). Among inhibited children, the rates of anxiety disorders had increased markedly from baseline to follow-up. The emergence of multiple anxiety disorders, including avoidant disorder, agoraphobia, and SAD in children who did not have these diagnoses at baseline, was also significantly greater for the inhibited compared with the noninhibited children. All children with "pathological" anxiety—that is, multiple (≥ 2) anxiety disorders—were observed to have behavioral inhibition. These data support the hypothesis of a developmental progression of an anxiety diathesis from behavioral inhibition to overanxious, phobic, and avoidant disorders in early childhood to SAD and finally agoraphobia in later childhood.

Family studies have supported these findings. Rosenbaum et al. (1988) reported that the rates of BI in children of probands with panic disorder and agoraphobia (PDAG), with or without comorbid major depression disorder (MDD), were significantly higher than in the group without PDAG. There was a progressively increased risk for BI in the offspring of a comparison group of control parents without MDD (15.4%), to parents with MDD (50%), comorbid PDAG and MDD (70%), and PDAG alone (84.6%).

Children with behavioral inhibition have higher rates of both anxiety and nonanxiety disorders than children without BI (Rosenbaum et al. 1993). Further work from this group (Biederman et al. 1990) demonstrated that children of parents with PDAG were at increased risk for childhood anxiety disorders and that the risk for multiple (≥ 2) anxiety disorders fell exclusively among those children with BI compared with those without BI. These findings were true for the children of parents in treatment for anxiety disorders (22% vs. 0%) as well as for children ascertained from a nonclinical population (18% vs. 0%).

Parents of children with BI are at increased risk for multiple anxiety disorders during adulthood, a history of anxiety disorders during childhood, and anxiety difficulties that persist from childhood to adulthood. In a nonclinically derived population, parents of inhibited children compared with those of uninhibited children or normal control subjects had elevated rates of social phobia, childhood avoidant disorder, and OAD (Rosenbaum et al. 1991), supporting the hypothesis that BI in children is linked to the familial predisposition to anxiety disorder. Parents of behaviorally inhibited children who also have an anxiety disorder were more likely to have multiple anxiety disorders than the parents of children with BI alone or those without BI or anxiety disorders (Rosenbaum et al. 1992). This finding supports the hypothesis that the presence of BI with an anxiety disorder may be a more severe manifestation of a diathesis for anxiety and further suggests that, although the presence of BI in a child may be an early manifestation of or may predispose to the development of an anxiety disorder, this may be more likely in the presence of high familial loading for anxiety. Thus, BI may represent a general anxiety proneness, with the specific syndrome that develops being determined by a number of genetic, familial, or psychosocial and psychological factors. The hypothesis of a diathesis of anxiety proneness corresponds to Torgersen's (1983) finding that identical twins of probands with panic disorder were concordant for anxiety symptoms, but not specifically for panic disorder.

Not all children remain behaviorally inhibited over time (Hirshfeld et al. 1992). Two phenotypic presentations of BI have been hypothesized based on research findings: a "stable BI" phenotype, which is associated with behavioral inhibition at least through age 7 and which is characterized by a high and stable heart rate and elevated rates of anxiety disorders in the parents, and an "unstable BI" phenotype, which is not persistent and which is less strongly associated with parental psychopathology. The association between

BI and the development of anxiety disorders over time may be stronger in children who exhibit stable BI.

Though clearly a risk factor for anxiety difficulties, the presence of BI does not ensure the development of psychopathology. Seventy percent of behaviorally inhibited children are free of anxiety disorders (Biederman et al. 1990), which suggests that other factors that are influencing the emergence of anxiety disorders may be critical as well. At present it is not clear whether BI is an independent risk factor for childhood-onset anxiety disorder or an added risk factor in children already at risk due to familial panic disorder and agoraphobia. Work is underway with a larger sample of children to better address these issues (Rosenbaum et al. 1993).

Separation Anxiety Disorder and School Refusal

Many follow-up studies of children with SAD predate DSM-III classification and do not distinguish between separation anxiety and school refusal. These studies primarily describe the course and prognosis of children with school refusal and do not apply systematic diagnostic assessments, which would permit more refined analysis. School refusal secondary to anxiety tends to fall into two categories: a separation anxiety type, which is more predominant in girls, and a phobic type, which is more predominant in boys (Last et al. 1987b). About 80% of cases of school refusal may be due to separation anxiety (Gittelman and Klein 1984); because the two have been linked in many studies, we will present follow-ups on school refusal in this section.

Children with school refusal are more likely to develop work phobia, employment difficulties, and social impairment (Coolidge et al. 1964; Waldron 1976). Follow-up studies of previously hospitalized school-phobic children 2–18 years after discharge report that 22%–100% of patients continue to experience significant anxiety symptoms, and many continue to require treatment (Boreham 1983; Roberts 1975; Warren 1965; Weiss and Burke 1970).

Outpatient studies of children with school phobia report a significant number of overall adjustment problems in children at fol-

low-up, including poor school attendance and interpersonal difficulties, with better outcomes generally in younger children
(Coolidge et al. 1964; Flakierska et al. 1988; Miller et al. 1972;
Rodriguez et al. 1959; Waldron 1976). In one general population
study of school phobia in Japan, half of a sample of school-phobic
children were still frequently absent from school at 1-year follow-up
(Ono 1972).

In an ongoing study of adults treated for school refusal as children (Klein and Last 1989), overall rates of anxiety disorders in
those children with school refusal have not differed from overall
rates of anxiety disorders in control subjects, although a significantly
greater rate of agoraphobia with panic disorder was noted in the
adults who had a history of separation anxiety. The prevalence of
social phobia was two times greater in those individuals with school
refusal, but this difference was not statistically significant. The rate
of major depression has not differed significantly between probands
and control subjects, although more depressive disorders have developed among probands (31% vs. 18%).

In a small follow-up study, Cantwell and Baker (1989) report
that separation anxiety disorder may be relatively more unstable
than other childhood anxiety disorders, noting a 44% recovery rate
in their 4-year follow-up of a subgroup of nine children initially
diagnosed with SAD. All of the children had received treatment,
which may have contributed to the high remission rate. Of those
who remained ill, only one (11%) still met criteria for separation
anxiety, whereas the others exhibited OAD and/or disruptive disorder. Their findings are consistent with the hypothesis that SAD
may be an early manifestation of an anxiety diathesis that is variably
expressed over time.

Treatment

Three treatment modalities—behavior therapy, pharmacotherapy,
and psychodynamic psychotherapy, either alone or in combination—have been reported effective in treatment of SAD and school
phobia. In one study, Blagg and Yule (1984) compared the relative
efficacies of behavioral therapy, hospitalization, and home tuition
with psychotherapy for treatment of school phobia. After 1 year,
93% of the behavioral therapy group, 37% of the hospital-treated

group, and 10% of the home tuition and psychotherapy group were doing well. The behavior therapy approach was also less costly and time intensive, although lack of random patient assignment in this study hampers interpretation of its study results.

Since the early benchmark study (Gittelman-Klein and Klein 1971) demonstrating the effectiveness of imipramine for school phobia, there have been several double-blind, placebo-controlled studies of the use of antidepressants to treat school absenteeism or SAD. The original study by Gittleman-Klein and Klein (1971, 1973) of 35 psychotherapy-resistant children with school absenteeism (93% of whom also had SAD) found that treatment with imipramine (100–200 mg/day) versus placebo for 6 weeks was superior in facilitating return to school, reducing anxiety and fear, and diminishing somatic symptoms regardless of the presence or absence of depression. However, in a later study, R. G. Klein et al. (1992) found no effect for imipramine (mean daily dose of 150 mg for 6 weeks) in 20 children with SAD who failed to respond to a 1-month trial of behavioral therapy. A double-blind study of the effectiveness of low-dose (40–75 mg/day) clomipramine in 27 school-phobic subjects did not find it superior to placebo for anxiety, although depressive symptoms were reduced (Berney et al. 1981). Bernstein et al. (1990) evaluated 24 children with school phobia and found that nonsignificant trends toward imipramine and alprazolam were more effective than placebo for treatment of anxiety and depressive symptoms.

Although three of the four studies did not clearly support the efficacy of tricyclic antidepressants (TCAs) for SAD and school phobia, the studies suffered from a variety of methodological limitations, including small sample size, failure to exclude patients with depression or other comorbidity, and the low doses used in the study of clomipramine. Klein and Last's (1989) ongoing double-blind comparison of the efficacy of behavioral therapy with placebo to that of behavioral therapy with imipramine in a group of nondepressed children with separation anxiety or school phobia may provide more information on the relative benefits of behavior therapy and TCAs for the treatment of these syndromes.

Benzodiazepines have also been used to treat school absenteeism. In one small double-blind, placebo-controlled study of alpra-

zolam (1–3 mg/day), school attendance improved in the six alpra-
zolam-treated subjects ages 9–17 (Bernstein et al. 1990). Open case
series of clonazepam (Biederman 1987), alprazolam (Kutcher et al.
1992), and chlordiazepoxide (Kraft et al. 1965) in children with
school absenteeism and SAD have also yielded encouraging results,
although evidence for the efficacy of the benzodiazepines in treating
SAD or school absenteeism remains suggestive and awaits further
systematic study.

Panic Disorder

There is relatively little reported information on the outcome of
childhood-onset panic disorder. Herman et al. (1981) examined
Mayo clinic records over a 25-year period and found 34 children
diagnosed with hyperventilation syndrome and symptoms suggestive of panic attacks. When these individuals were contacted for
follow-up information, many reported chronic anxiety, suggesting
that hyperventilation syndrome may represent a childhood anxiety
disorder or precursor of adult anxiety disorders.

Treatment
Cognitive and behavioral treatment for panic disorder in children
has been reported effective in open trials, but has not yet been
subject to systematic clinical trials. Reports on psychopharmacological treatment of childhood panic disorder are also comprised of
uncontrolled clinical trials and suggest that the antidepressants imipramine or desipramine (Black and Robbins 1990; Black et al.
1990) and the benzodiazepines alprazolam (Ballenger et al. 1989)
and clonazepam (Biederman 1987) can be helpful in eliminating
panic symptoms. Kutcher et al. (1992) are currently obtaining encouraging results in an ongoing double-blind, placebo-controlled
study of clonazepam in adolescents with panic disorder.

Overanxious Disorder

OAD is relatively common in clinic samples, with prevalence rates
ranging from 13%–51% (Last and Perrin 1993; Last et al. 1992;

Strauss et al. 1988). Relatively little is known about the natural history of OAD because it appeared as a diagnostic category for the first time in DSM-III. Cantwell and Baker (1989) found that only 25% of children initially diagnosed with OAD were psychiatrically well at 4-year follow-up, with some children going on to develop avoidant disorder, disruptive disorder, and major depression. A naturalistic study of 275 children between the ages of 6 and 19 noted that of the 14% who had a history of anxiety disorder, 82% met criteria for OAD, with a mean age at onset of 10 years and a mean duration of episode of 4.5 years (Keller et al. 1992).

Whether OAD is a discrete disorder remains controversial. OAD may be a prodromal state for the development of other anxiety disorders, although it often occurs after the development of other disorders. Ninety percent of children with panic disorder and OAD in one study developed OAD before the onset of panic (Last et al. 1992).

Treatment

Clinical treatment of OAD has generally involved teaching crisis management skills, desensitization methods for specific anxiety-provoking situations, and family counseling and education (Husain and Kashani 1992). One small study (Kane and Kendall 1989) of four children with OAD treated with cognitive-behavioral therapy demonstrated improvement acutely and at 3- and 6-month follow-up. Clonazepam has been reported to be helpful in a child with OAD (Biederman 1987), as was alprazolam in a small series of OAD patients treated with 0.5–1.5 mg/day (Simeon and Ferguson 1987). However, in a 4-week, double-blind, placebo-controlled study of 21 children (ages 8–16 years) with OAD, alprazolam showed a slightly greater (but nonsignificant) mean clinical global improvement compared with placebo (Simeon et al. 1992), although relatively low doses (0.5–3.5 mg/day, average daily dose = 1.6 mg) may have been inadequate to demonstrate a full effect. Treatment with buspirone, an azapirone, has been noted to be effective in children and adolescents (Allen et al. 1993) and was also found to reduce anxiety within 6 weeks in a pilot study of adolescents with OAD who were treated with 15–30 mg/day (Kutcher et al. 1992).

Avoidant Disorder and Social Phobia

The natural history of avoidant disorder has not been well studied, but available information suggests it generally has a chronic, stable course. Cantwell and Baker (1989) noted that, although only 29% of children initially diagnosed with avoidant disorder still had the disorder 4 years later, most (64%) were still psychiatrically ill. Although avoidant disorder may be a precursor to avoidant personality disorder or social phobia in adults, there is no definitive data yet to establish this relationship.

The onset of social phobia is typically in childhood or adolescence (Liebowitz et al. 1985; Turner et al. 1986). The mean number of years of social distress in one study (Turner et al. 1986) was 20.9 years, with a range of 5–46 years, suggesting that social anxiety during childhood is likely to be chronic and unremitting in nature.

Treatment

Although there has been little empirical study of cognitive-behavioral therapy for children specifically identified as meeting diagnostic criteria for avoidant disorder or social phobia, several studies have focused on children identified as shy, socially isolated or withdrawn, or peer neglected. A number of cognitive-behavioral interventions—including play therapy, behavior modification, cognitive therapy, social skills training, modeling, and family therapy—have been reported effective in the treatment of avoidant disorder (Husain and Kashani 1992). In one small study, avoidant children with long-standing social fears treated in a participant modeling format demonstrated reductions in fears and retained effectiveness of treatment at 6-month follow-up (Matson 1981). Preliminary data suggest that a 12-week group cognitive-behavioral treatment program, including social skills training and exposure, is effective for socially phobic adolescents (Albano et al. 1992). Strain and Fox (1981) have suggested that treatments for social isolation that incorporate a child's peers (i.e., peer-mediated approaches) may be superior to adult-mediated approaches because the former may facilitate changes in both social behavior and peer acceptance. Support for this comes from a study by Furman et al. (1979) demonstrating that socially withdrawn preschoolers given the opportunity to interact with sociable playmates in free-play sessions showed increased peer interaction compared with no-treatment control subjects.

Alprazolam was reported effective in case studies for the treatment of avoidant disorder (Simeon and Ferguson 1987), although a small double-blind, placebo-controlled study demonstrated only a trend toward more effectiveness of low-dose alprazolam (1.6 mg/day) than placebo (Simeon et al. 1992).

Phobic Disorders

Childhood fears and phobias generally represent transient developmental phenomena that disappear with time in the majority of children; however, a subset of children with simple phobias continue to have persistent symptoms. Although a number of studies conclude that mild fears are quite common in children of all ages (Silverman and Nelles 1990), recent studies employing DSM-III and DSM-III-R criteria have estimated the prevalence rate of simple phobias in children to be approximately 2%–3% (Anderson et al. 1987; Bird et al. 1988).

Although some report that the foci of fears change as children mature, with fears of doctors, injections, darkness, and strangers generally short-lived and declining with age and fears of animals, heights, storms, enclosed places, and social situations persisting (Agras et al. 1969), Ollendick et al. (1989) observed that common fears were remarkably consistent throughout different age, gender, and cultural groups studied and interpreted the consistency across different age groups as evidence for the persistence of childhood fears.

Agras et al. (1972) followed the simple phobias of 10 children and 20 adults over 5 years and reported that all of the children but only 43% of the adults improved. None of the children or adults received treatment for their phobic condition during the 5-year period. However, Ollendick (1979) has pointed out that none of the phobic children or adolescents were asymptomatic at follow-up, demonstrating a chronic course for some phobic individuals from childhood into the adult years.

Treatment

Simple phobias are most commonly treated with behavior therapy. In one study of anxious children and adolescents (ages 6–15), Miller et al. (1972) compared imaginal desensitization, psychotherapy, and waiting-list control conditions in the treatment of a variety of fears: school, dark, dogs, storms, heights, germs, physical injury, elevators, nakedness, and deep water. Both treatment groups, but not those on the waiting list, experienced significant improvement, and there was no difference between active treatments. At 2-year follow-up, 80% of the children were either symptom-free or significantly improved, although 7% continued to display severe phobias despite treatment.

Posttraumatic Stress Disorder

PTSD is seen frequently in clinic settings; a 9% prevalence rate has been noted in urban young adults (Breslau et al. 1991). Sexual abuse is one of the most common causes of PTSD in children. Over 40% of sexually abused children have been found to meet full diagnostic criteria for PTSD (McLeer et al. 1992).

The nature of the trauma affects the outcome over time for afflicted children (Terr 1991). When human accountability is tied to the stressor or the event is intentional or perpetrated by authority figures close to the child (e.g., sexual or physical abuse), its impact may be more severe and may cause long-lasting personality changes, including changes in the ability to trust or establish meaningful relationships (Herman 1992). Traumatic events before age 11 are three times more likely to result in PTSD, suggesting that children may be more sensitive to trauma than adolescents or adults (Davidson and Smith 1990). Studies suggest that PTSD symptomatology can continue for long periods of time. Pynoos et al. (1987) found that almost 60% of exposed children continued to meet full criteria for PTSD 1 month after a schoolyard sniper attack. Kinzie et al. (1989) found that 48% of adolescent Cambodian survivors of political atrocities had PTSD symptoms and persistent symptoms of depression and anxiety at 10-year follow-up.

Treatment

A variety of cognitive-behavioral and psychodynamic therapies for PTSD in adults (which have been reviewed by Solomon et al. 1992) may be useful for enhancing coping skills and treating traumatized children, although there are no published studies. Pharmacological treatment for children, as for adults, is often focused on treatment of comorbid anxiety or mood disorders, although there is little available systematic outcome data. In an open trial of 11 traumatized children (mean age 8.5 years), administration of the beta-blocker propranolol reduced the aggressiveness and anxiety associated with acute PTSD, an effect that reversed on drug discontinuation (Famularo et al. 1988). Clonidine has been reported to reduce startle reactions and avoidant behaviors in children with PTSD (Kinzie and Leung 1989).

▼ Summary

The available evidence points to a chronic course for many children who suffer from anxiety disorders. A substantial proportion of children continue to suffer anxiety difficulties despite treatment. Studies in animals and humans suggest that BI and excessive shyness during childhood may be early manifestations of a diathesis for the development of anxiety and mood disturbance during childhood and may serve as risk factors for the development of anxiety disorders over time. However, constitutional differences in temperament may be amplified or muted by environmental influences such as parental psychopathology or stress, suggesting that modifications in the psychosocial milieu, including treatment of parental psychopathology and education of parents regarding strategies for handling at-risk children, may modify the development of anxiety difficulties. For some children, early intervention with cognitive-behavioral, psychotherapeutic, or pharmacological therapies may improve acute function and reduce the impact of anxiety difficulties on self-esteem, social function, and school and work competence.

Although anxiety disorders are common in childhood, they often go unrecognized, and their potential long-term effects may not be fully appreciated. Increasing research on children at risk for anxiety difficulties and the proliferation of programs targeted to affected and at-risk children and adolescents should promote a greater recognition of this problem, increase research into the phenomenology and treatment of anxiety disorders in children, and improve acute and long-term outcome.

▼ References

Abe K, Masui T: Age-sex trends of phobic and anxiety symptoms. Br J Psychiatry 138:297–302, 1981

Abelson JL, Alessi NE: Discussion of "Child Panic Revisited." J Am Acad Child Adolesc Psychiatry 31:114–116, 1992

Agras S, Sylvester D, Oliveau D: The epidemiology of common fears and phobia. Compr Psychiatry 10:151–156, 1969

Agras WS, Chapin HN, Oliveau DC: The natural history of phobia. Arch Gen Psychiatry 26:315–317, 1972

Albano AM, Marten PA, Holt CS, et al: Cognitive-behavioral group treatment for social phobia in adolescents: a preliminary study. Paper presented at the World Congress of Behavior Therapy, Queensland, Australia, July, 1992

Allen AJ, Rapoport JL, Swedo SE: Psychopharmacologic treatment of childhood anxiety disorders. Child and Adolescent Psychiatric Clinics of North America 2:795–817, 1993

American Psychiatric Association: Diagnostic and Statistical Manual of Mental Disorders, 3rd Edition. Washington, DC, American Psychiatric Association, 1980

American Psychiatric Association: Diagnostic and Statistical Manual of Mental Disorders, 3rd Edition, Revised. Washington, DC, American Psychiatric Association, 1987

Anderson JC, Williams S, McGee R, et al: DSM-III disorders in preadolescent children. Arch Gen Psychiatry 44:69–76, 1987

Aronson TA, Logue CM: On the longitudinal course of panic disorder: developmental history and predictors of phobic complications. Compr Psychiatry 28:344–355, 1987

Ayuso JL, Alfonso S, Rivera A: Childhood separation anxiety and panic disorder: a comparative study. Prog Neuropsychopharmacol Biol Psychiatry 13:665–671, 1989

Ballenger JC, Carey DJ, Steele JJ, et al: Three cases of panic disorder with agoraphobia in children. Am J Psychiatry 146:922–925, 1989

Beidel DC: Psychophysiological assessment of anxious emotional states in children. J Abnorm Psychol 97:80–82, 1988

Berg I: School phobia in the children of agoraphobic women. Br J Psychiatry 128:86–89, 1976

Berg I, Butler A, Pritchard J: Psychiatric illness in the mothers of school phobic adolescents. Br J Psychiatry 125:466–467, 1974a

Berg I, Marks I, McGuire R, et al: School phobia and agoraphobia. Psychol Med 4:428–434, 1974b

Berkson J: Limitations of the application of fourfold table analysis to hospital data. Biometrics Bulletin 2:47–53, 1946

Berney T, Kolvin I, Bhate SR, et al: School phobia: a therapeutic trial with clomipramine and short-term outcome. Br J Psychiatry 138:110–118, 1981

Bernstein GA, Borchardt CM: Anxiety disorders of childhood and adolescence: a critical review. J Am Acad Child Adolesc Psychiatry 30:519–532, 1991

Bernstein GA, Garfinkel BD, Borchardt CM: Comparative studies of pharmacotherapy for school refusal. J Am Acad Child Adolesc Psychiatry 29:773–781, 1990

Biederman J: Clonazepam in the treatment of prepubertal children with panic-like symptoms. J Clin Psychiatry 48 (suppl 10):38–41, 1987

Biederman J, Rosenbaum JF, Hirshfeld DR, et al: Psychiatric correlates of behavioral inhibition in young children of parents with and without psychiatric disorders. Arch Gen Psychiatry 47:21–26, 1990

Biederman J, Rosenbaum JF, Bolduc-Murphy EA, et al: A three year follow-up of children with and without behavioral inhibition in patients with attention deficit disorder: a controlled study. J Am Acad Child Adolesc Psychiatry 32:814–821, 1993

Bird HR, Canino G, Rubio-Stipee M, et al: Estimates of the prevalence of childhood maladjustment in a community survey in Puerto Rico. Arch Gen Psychiatry 45:1120–1126, 1988

Black B, Robbins DR: Panic disorder in children and adolescents. J Am Acad Child Adolesc Psychiatry 29:36–44, 1990

Black B, Uhde TW, Robbins DR: Reply to DF Klein, RG Klein: does panic disorder exist in children? (letter) J Am Acad Child Adolesc Psychiatry 29:834–835, 1990

Blagg NR, Yule W: The behavioral treatment of school refusal—comparative study. Behav Res Ther 22:119–127, 1984

Bondareff W, Mountjoy CQ: Number of neurons in the nucleus locus ceruleus in demented and nondemented patients: rapid estimation and correlated parameters. Neurobiol Aging 7:297–300, 1986

Boreham J: A follow-up study of 54 persistent school refusers. Association for Child Psychology and Psychiatry News 15:8–14, 1983

Breier A, Charney DS, Heninger JR: Major depression in patients with agoraphobia and panic disorder. Arch Gen Psychiatry 31:1129–1135, 1984

Breslau N, Davis G, Andreski P, et al: Traumatic events and post traumatic stress disorder in an urban population of young adults. Arch Gen Psychiatry 48:216–222, 1991

Cantwell DP, Baker L: Stability and natural history of DSM-III childhood diagnoses. J Am Acad Child Adolesc Psychiatry 28:691–700, 1989

Charney DS, Woods SW, Nagy LM, et al: Noradrenergic function in panic disorder. J Clin Psychiatry 51(suppl A):5–11, 1990

Coolidge JC, Brodie RD, Feeney B: A ten year follow up study of sixty six school children. Am J Orthopsychiatry 34:675–684, 1964

Crowe RR, Noyes R, Pauls DL, et al: A family study of panic disorder. Arch Gen Psychiatry 40:1065–1069, 1983

Davidson S, Smith R: Traumatic experiences in psychiatric outpatients. Journal of Traumatic Stress Studies 3:459–475, 1990

Deltito JA, Perugi G, Maremmani I, et al: The importance of separation anxiety in the differentiation of panic disorder from agoraphobia. Psychiatr Dev 3:227–236, 1986

Earls F: The prevalence of behavior problems in three year old children: a cross-cultural replication. Arch Gen Psychiatry 37:1153–1156, 1980

Famularo R, Kinscherff R, Fenton T: Propranolol treatment for childhood post traumatic stress disorder, acute type: a pilot study. Am J Dis Child 142:1244–1247, 1988

Feldman RD, Limbird LE, Nadeau J, et al: Alterations in leukocyte beta receptor affinity with aging: a potential explanation for altered beta-adrenergic sensitivity in the elderly. N Engl J Med 310:815–819, 1984

Fischer M, Rolf JE, Hasazi JE, et al: Follow-up of a preschool epidemiological sample: cross-age continuities and predictions of later adjustment with internalizing and externalizing dimensions of behavior. Child Dev 55:137–150, 1984

Flakierska N, Lindstrom M, Gillberg C: School refusal: a 15–20 year follow-up study of 35 Swedish urban children. Br J Psychiatry 152:834–837, 1988

Furman W, Rahe DF, Hartup WW: Rehabilitation of socially withdrawn preschool children through mixed-age and same-age socialization. Child Dev 50:915–922, 1979

Gittelman-Klein R: Psychiatric characteristics of the relatives of school phobic children, in Mental Health in Children, Vol 1. Edited by Sankar DVS. New York, PJD, 1975

Gittelman-Klein R, Klein DF: Controlled imipramine treatment of school phobia. Arch Gen Psychiatry 25:204–207, 1971

Gittelman-Klein R, Klein DF: School phobia: diagnostic considerations in the light of imipramine effects. J Nerv Ment Dis 156:199–215, 1973

Gittelman-Klein R, Klein DF: Relationship between separation anxiety and panic and agoraphobic disorders. Psychopathology 17:56–65, 1984

Herman JL: Complex PTSD: a syndrome in survivors of prolonged and repeated trauma. Journal of Traumatic Stress 5:377–391, 1992

Herman S, Stickler G, Lucas A: Hyperventilation syndrome in children and adolescents: long-term follow-up. Pediatrics 67:183–187, 1981

Hirshfeld DR, Rosenbaum JF, Biederman J, et al: Stable behavioral inhibition and its association with anxiety disorder patients with attention deficit disorder: a controlled study. J Am Acad Child Adolesc Psychiatry 31:103–111, 1992

Husain SA, Kashani JH: Anxiety Disorders in Children and Adolescents. Washington, DC, American Psychiatric Press, 1992

Kagan J, Snidman N: Infant predictors of inhibited and uninhibited profiles. Psychological Sciences 2:40–44, 1991

Kagan J, Reznick JS, Snidman N: Biological bases of childhood shyness. Science 240:167–171, 1988

Kane MT, Kendall PC: Anxiety disorders in children: a multiple-baseline evaluation of a cognitive-behavioral treatment. Behavior Therapy 20:499–508, 1989

Kashani JH, Orvaschel H: Anxiety disorders in mid-adolescence: a community sample. Am J Psychiatry 145:960–964, 1988

Kastrup M: Psychic disorders among preschool children in a geographically delimited area of Aarhus County, Denmark. Acta Psychiatr Scand 54:29–42, 1976

Keller MB, Lavori PW, Wunder J, et al: Chronic course of anxiety disorders in children and adolescents. J Am Acad Child Adolesc Psychiatry 31:595–599, 1992

Kimura F, Nakamura S: Locus coeruleus neurons in the neonatal rat: electrical activity and responses to sensory stimulation. Developing Brain Research 23:301–305, 1985

Kimura F, Nakamura S: Post-natal development of δ-adrenoceptor-mediated auto inhibition in the locus coeruleus. Developing Brain Research 35:21–26, 1987

Kinzie JD, Leung P: Clonidine in Cambodian patients with posttraumatic stress disorder. J Nerv Ment Dis 177:546–550, 1989

Kinzie JD, Sack W, Angell R, et al: A three year follow-up of Cambodian young people traumatized as children. J Am Acad Child Adolesc Psychiatry 28:501–504, 1989

Klein DF: Delineation of two drug responsive anxiety syndromes. Psychopharmacologia 5:397–408, 1964

Klein DF: Psychopharmacologic treatment of panic disorder. Psychosomatics 25(suppl):32–36, 1984

Klein DF, Last CG: Anxiety Disorders in Children. Newbury Park, CA, Sage Publications, 1989

Klein DF, Mannuzza S, Chapman T, et al: Child panic revisited. J Am Acad Child Adolesc Psychiatry 31:112–116, 1992

Klein RG, Koplewicz HS, Kanner A: Imipramine treatment of children with separation anxiety disorder. J Am Acad Child Adolesc Psychiatry 31:21–28, 1992

Kraft IA, Ardali C, Duffy JH, et al: A clinical study of chlordiazepoxide used in psychiatric disorders of children. International Journal of Neuropsychiatry 1:433–437, 1965

Kutcher SP, Reiter S, Gardner DM, et al: The pharmacotherapy of anxiety disorders in children and adolescents. Psychiatr Clin North Am 15:41–67, 1992

Lapouse R, Monk MA: An epidemiologic study of behavior characteristics in children. Am J Public Health 48:1134–1144, 1958

Last CG, Perrin S: Anxiety disorders in African-American and white children. J Abnorm Child Psychol 21:153–164, 1993

Last CG, Strauss CC: School refusal in anxiety-disordered children and adolescents. J Am Acad Child Adolesc Psychiatry 29:31–35, 1990

Last CG, Strauss CC, Francis G: Comorbidity among childhood anxiety disorders. J Nerv Ment Dis 175:726–730, 1987a

Last CG, Francis G, Hersen M, et al: Separation anxiety and school phobia: a comparison using DSM-III criteria. Am J Psychiatry 144:653–657, 1987b

Last CG, Hersen M, Kazdin A, et al: Psychiatric illness in the mothers of anxious children. Am J Psychiatry 144:1580–1583, 1987c

Last CG, Hersen M, Kazdin A, et al: Anxiety disorders in children and their families. Arch Gen Psychiatry 148:928–934, 1991

Last CG, Perrin S, Hersen M, et al: DSM-III-R anxiety disorders in children: sociodemographic and clinical characteristics. J Am Acad Child Adolesc Psychiatry 31:1070–1076, 1992

Laurent J, Landau S, Stark KD: Conditional probabilities in the diagnosis of depressive and anxiety disorders in children. School Psychology Review 22:98–114, 1993

Liebowitz MR, Gorman JM, Fyer AJ, et al: Social phobia. Arch Gen Psychiatry 42:729–736, 1985

Markowitz JS, Weissman MM, Ouellette R, et al: Quality of life in panic disorder. Arch Gen Psychiatry 46:984–992, 1989

Matson JL: Assessment and treatment of clinical fears in mentally retarded children. J Appl Behav Anal 14:287–293, 1981

McGee R, Feehan M, Williams S, et al: DSM-III disorders in a large sample of adolescents. J Am Acad Child Adolesc Psychiatry 29:611–619, 1990

McLeer SV, Deblinger E, Henry D, et al: Sexually abused children at high risk for post-traumatic stress disorder. J Am Acad Child Adolesc Psychiatry 31:875–879, 1992

Miller LC, Barrett CL, Hampe E, et al: Comparison of reciprocal inhibition, psychotherapy and waiting list control. J Abnorm Psychol 79:269–279, 1972

Munir K, Biederman J, Knee D: Psychiatric comorbidity in patients with attention deficit disorder: a controlled study. J Am Acad Child Adolesc Psychiatry 26:844–848, 1987

Nelles WB, Barlow DH: Do children panic? Clinical Psychology Review 8:359–372, 1988

Ollendick TH: Fear reduction techniques with children, in Progress in Behavior Modification, Vol 18. Edited by Hersen M, Eisler RM, Miller PM. New York, Academic Press, 1979, pp 127–168

Ollendick TH, King NJ, Frary RB: Fears in children and adolescents: reliability and generalizability across gender, age and nationality. Behav Res Ther 27:19–26, 1989

Olpe HR, Steinmann MW: Age related decline in the activity of noradrenergic neurons of the rat locus coeruleus. Brain Res 251:174–176, 1982

Ono O: Basic studies in school phobia: an investigation in a local area (Kagawa Prefecture). Japanese Journal of Child Psychiatry 13:249–260, 1972

Otto MW, Pollack MH, Rosenbaum JF, et al: Childhood history of anxiety in adults with panic disorder: association with anxiety sensitivity and comorbidity. Harvard Review of Psychiatry 1:288–293, 1994

Perugi G, Deltito J, Sorinani A, et al: Relationships between panic disorder and separation anxiety with school phobia. Compr Psychiatry 29:98–107, 1988

Pollack MH, Otto MW, Rosenbaum JF, et al: Longitudinal course of panic disorder: findings from the Massachusetts General Hospital Naturalistic Study. J Clin Psychiatry 51:12–16, 1990

Pollack MH, Otto MW, Rosenbaum JF, et al: Personality disorders in patients with panic disorder: association with childhood anxiety disorders, early trauma, comorbidity, and chronicity. Compr Psychiatry 33:78–83, 1992

Popper CW: Psychopharmacologic treatment of anxiety disorders in adolescents and children. J Clin Psychiatry 54:52–63, 1993

Pynoos RS, Frederick C, Nader K, et al: Life threat and post traumatic stress in school age children. Arch Gen Psychiatry 44:1057–1063, 1987

Raskin M, Peek HVS, Dickman W, et al: Panic and generalized anxiety disorders, developmental antecedents, and precipitants. Arch Gen Psychiatry 39:687–689, 1982

Reiss S, Peterson RA, Gursky M, et al: Anxiety sensitivity, anxiety frequency and the prediction of fearfulness. Behav Res Ther 24:1–8, 1986

Richman N, Stevenson JE, Graham PJ: Prevalence of behavior problems in three-year old children: an epidemiologic study in a London borough. J Child Psychol Psychiatry 16:277–287, 1975

Roberts M: Persistent school refusal among children and adolescents, in Life History Research in Psychopathology, Vol 4. Edited by Wirt DR, Winokur G, Roff M. Minneapolis, University of Minnesota Press, 1975, pp 79–108

Robinson DS, Davis JM, Nies A, et al: Aging monoamines and monoamine-oxidase levels. Lancet 1:290–291, 1972

Rodriguez A, Rodriguez M, Eisenberg L: The outcome of school phobia: a follow-up study based on 41 cases. Am J Psychiatry 116:540–544, 1959

Rosenbaum JF, Biederman J, Gersten M, et al: Behavioral inhibition in children of parents with panic disorder and agoraphobia. Arch Gen Psychiatry 45:463–470, 1988

Rosenbaum JF, Biederman J, Hirshfeld DR, et al: Further evidence of an association between behavioral inhibition and anxiety disorders: results from a family study of children from a non-clinical sample. J Psychiatr Res 25:49–65, 1991

Rosenbaum JF, Biederman J, Bolduc EA, et al: Comorbidity in parental anxiety disorders as risk for childhood-onset anxiety in inhibited children. Am J Psychiatry 149:475–481, 1992

Rosenbaum JF, Biederman J, Bolduc-Murphy EA, et al: Behavioral inhibition in childhood: a risk factor for anxiety disorders. Harvard Review of Psychiatry 1:2–16, 1993

Rosenblum LA, Coplan JD, Friedman S, et al: Adverse early experiences affect noradrenergic and serotonergic functioning in adult primates. Biol Psychiatry 35:221–227, 1994

Rutter M, Sandberg S: Epidemiology of child psychiatric disorder: methodological issues and some substantive findings. Child Psychiatry Hum Dev 15:209–233, 1985

Silverman WK, Nelles WB: Simple phobia in childhood, in Handbook of Child and Adult Psychopathology: A Longitudinal Perspective. Edited by Hersen M, Last CG. New York, Pergamon, 1990, pp 183–196

Simeon J , Ferguson B: Alprazolam effects in children with anxiety disorder. Can J Psychiatry 32:570–574, 1987

Simeon JC, Ferguson B, Nott V, et al: Clinical, cognitive, and neurophysiological effects of alprazolam in children and adolescents with overanxious and avoidant disorders. J Am Acad Child Adolesc Psychiatry 31:29–33, 1992

Solomon S, Gerritz L, Muff A: Efficacy of treatments for post traumatic stress disorder: an empirical review. JAMA 268:633–638, 1992

Strain PS, Fox JE: Peers as therapeutic agents for isolate classmates, in Advances in Clinical Child Psychology, Vol IV. Edited by Kasden AE, Lahey BB. New York, Plenum, 1981, pp 167–198

Strauss CC, Lahey EB, Frick P, et al: Peer social status of children with anxiety disorders. J Consult Clin Psychol 56:137–141, 1988

Suomi SJ: Anxiety-like disorders in young nonhuman primates, in Anxiety Disorders of Childhood. Edited by Gittelman R. New York, Guilford, 1986, pp 1–23

Terr LC: Childhood traumas: an outline and overview. Am J Psychiatry 148:10–19, 1991

Thyer BA, Parris RT, Curtis GC, et al: Ages of onset of DSM-III anxiety disorders. Compr Psychiatry 26:113–122, 1985

Torgersen S: Genetic factors in anxiety disorders. Arch Gen Psychiatry 40:1085–1089, 1983

Turner SM, Beidel DC, Dancu CV, et al: Psychopathology of social phobia and comparison to avoidant personality disorder. J Abnorm Psychol 95:389–394, 1986

Turner SM, Beidel DC, Costello A: Psychopathology in offspring of anxiety disorder patients. J Consult Clin Psychol 55:229–235, 1987

Tyrer P, Tyrer S: School refusal, truancy, and adult neurotic illness. Psychol Med 4:416–421, 1974

von Korff MR, Eaton WW, Keyl PM: The epidemiology of panic attacks and panic disorder: results of three community surveys. Am J Epidemiol 122:970–981, 1985

Waldron S: The significance of childhood neurosis for adult mental health: a follow-up study. Am J Psychiatry 133:532–538, 1976

Warren W: A study of adolescent psychiatric in-patients and the outcome six or more years later, II: the follow-up study. J Child Psychol Psychiatry 6:141–160, 1965

Weiss M, Burke A: A 5- to 10-year follow-up of hospitalized school phobic children and adolescents. Am J Orthopsychiatry 40:672–676, 1970

Weissman MM, Leckman JF, Merikangas KR, et al: Depression and anxiety disorders in parents and children. Arch Gen Psychiatry 41:845–852, 1984

Weissman MM, Klerman GL, Markowitz JS, et al: Suicidal ideation and suicide attempts in panic disorder and attacks. N Engl J Med 321:1209–1214, 1989

Werry JS, Quay HC: The prevalence of behavior symptoms in younger elementary school children. Am J Orthopsychiatry 41:136–143, 1971

Williams JT, Marshall KC: Membrane properties in adrenergic response in locus coeruleus neurons in young rats. J Neurosci 7:3687–3694, 1987

Chapter 8

Obsessive-Compulsive Disorder

**Joanna Pleeter,
Marge C. Lenane, M.S.W., and
Henrietta L. Leonard, M.D.**

Obsessive-compulsive disorder (OCD) has been described in adults for centuries, with early references to scrupulosity (one form of obsessions) in religious writings. In 1522, Ignatius Loyola confessed his scrupulosity in religious writings: "I feel some uneasiness on the subject [whether or not I have sinned], inasmuch as I doubt and yet do not doubt. This is probably a scruple . . ." (cited in Suess and Halpern 1989, p. 311). Obsessions are also referred to in historic Judaic writings. Interestingly, the purifying ceremony, Hatarat Nedarim, which allows for renunciation of forgotten vows, vows taken in a dreamlike state, and even vows of which the person is still aware and yet unable to fulfill, has been used on occasion to relieve the guilt of the worried OCD patient (Suess and Halpern 1989).

In the 17th century, Shakespeare described Lady Macbeth's compulsive handwashing. Freud (1909/1955) published the psychoanalysis of a patient with "obsessional neurosis" known as "The Rat Man," and theorized that pregenital sexual organization was the underlying cause of the "choice" symptom in this neurosis. Since that time, there have been numerous case reports of individuals with obsessions accompanied by ritualistic behaviors, who have been variously categorized as having obsessional neurosis, anancastic personality disorder, or obsessional personality.

OCD has been described in children as well as in adults. Pierre Janet (1903) described a 5-year-old child with symptoms of OCD and likened the obsessions to "mental tics." Kanner (1935; cited in Kanner 1962) reviewed the older reports on childhood OCD and emphasized the social isolation of these children. Berman (1942) described four cases of pediatric OCD with adult symptom profiles. Despert (1955) reported 68 pediatric cases of "obsessive-compulsive neurosis" and noted that the children were aware of the abnormality of their behavior. Just over 30 years ago, Judd (1965) described five children with OCD, and set out criteria that were quite similar to those of modern day DSM-III-R (American Psychiatric Association 1987). The Judd criteria suggested that the patient's obsessive-compulsive symptoms had to be the most prominent psychopathology and had to be severe enough to interfere with the child's everyday functioning.

▼ Definition

OCD is defined by DSM-III-R as an illness characterized by "recurrent obsessions or compulsions which are sufficiently severe to cause marked distress, be time-consuming, or which significantly interfere with the person's normal routine, occupational functioning, or usual social activities or relationships with others." Obsessions are recurrent and persistent thoughts, impulses, images, or ideas that are often senseless and intrusive. Compulsions are intended repetitive actions, which are acted out in response to obsessions. OCD was similarly defined by ICD-10 criteria (World Health Organization 1992) as requiring that "obsessive symptoms or compulsive acts must be present most days for at least 2 successive weeks and be a source of distress or interference activities." Interestingly, ICD-10 delineated OCD into subtypes that included predominantly obsessional thoughts, predominantly compulsive acts, mixed obsessional thoughts and acts, other obsessive-compulsive disorders, and an unspecified category.

Until recently, there were no standardized criteria for OCD, and this heterogeneous group of patients was simply labeled as "obsessional." This lack of early standardized diagnostic criteria has made it particularly difficult to review the early literature and to draw conclusions about the samples described in follow-up studies. Additionally, the absence of structured interviews and rating scales made systematic comparison difficult to interpret between baseline and follow-up status, both within and between samples. These issues are detailed later in the chapter.

▼ Phenomenology and Epidemiology

The specific obsessions and compulsions of children with OCD are essentially the same as those described in adults (Swedo et al. 1989; Thomsen and Mikkelsen 1991). In a large systematic study of 70 consecutive children and adolescents with OCD evaluated at the National Institute of Mental Health (NIMH), the most common obsessions included concerns about dirt or germs, worries about harm coming to self or loved ones, scrupulosity, and somatic preoccupations (Swedo et al. 1989). The most common rituals were excessive washing, repeating, checking, touching, ordering, counting, and hoarding. The illness is typically characterized by waxing and waning symptomatology and may be exacerbated by psychosocial stress. Interestingly, Rettew et al. (1992) reported that in 79 children and adolescents with OCD studied over an 8-year period (range 2–16 years), none of the patients maintained the same symptom constellation from baseline to follow-up. No discernible patterns with regard to any specific symptom or age could be found. The majority of patients had a variety of symptoms, which changed in both content and severity over time.

OCD in the pediatric age group is far more common than initially thought. Estimates of prevalence vary greatly, perhaps in part because of the secretiveness frequently exhibited by these children. In the Isle of Wight population survey of 2,000 10- and 11-year-olds, an 0.3% prevalence rate was reported (Rutter et al. 1970). Flament et al.'s (1988) epidemiological survey of 5,596 high school students reported weighted estimates of 1% (current) and 1.9% (lifetime) prevalences.

▼ Neurobiology and Treatment

Until recently, OCD was thought to be primarily a neurotic disorder, the manifestation of intrapsychic conflicts, and thus psychoanalysis was the primary treatment. In the last decade, with the explosion in neurobiological research, OCD has been approached from neurophysiological, neuroanatomic, and neuroimmunological viewpoints. The "serotonin hypothesis" of OCD was based on the success of serotonin reuptake inhibitors in treating OCD (Insel et al. 1985) and on challenge studies. More recently, it is clear that multiple neurotransmitters are likely involved, and there has been speculation that dopaminergic dysregulation may be implicated in the pathophysiology (Goodman et al. 1990; Swedo and Rapoport 1990). Systematic family studies suggest that in some OCD patients there may be genetic transmission of the illness (Lenane et al. 1990; Pauls et al. 1986). For a review of the neurobiology of OCD the reader is referred to Insel (1992).

OCD, for the most part, has been refractory to the more traditional psychodynamically oriented treatments. With the recent availability of the serotonin reuptake inhibitors (SRIs) and the development of new behavior therapy techniques, there has been a dramatic change in the treatment options and their efficacy for OCD. The SRIs, such as clomipramine, fluoxetine, sertraline, and fluvoxamine, have been effective in the treatment of OCD in adults (Jenike 1992). Of these, only clomipramine and fluoxetine have been systematically evaluated in children, and they have proven to be safe and effective for OCD in the pediatric age group (DeVeaugh-Geiss et al. 1992; Flament et al. 1985; Leonard et al. 1989; Riddle et al. 1992). Sertraline and fluvoxamine are under study in the younger age group and may prove to be similar to the other SRIs in terms of safety and efficacy. Long-term maintenance may be required for medication-responsive patients (Leonard et al. 1991). In a double-blind desipramine substitution study of long-term clomipramine-maintained patients, the majority (8 of 9) of the substituted patients relapsed, whereas only 2 of 11 nonsubstituted patients did. Clinically, even those patients on maintenance therapy had continued OCD symptoms with a waxing and waning course (Leonard et al. 1991).

Behavior therapy is considered one of the treatments of choice in children with OCD, although it has not been systematically studied in children (C.J. Berg et al. 1989). Exposure with response prevention (Marks 1987) is the specific approach and is applicable to the pediatric population (C.J. Berg et al. 1989a). In this treatment, the patient is exposed to a feared situation, and then the response (the ritual) is prevented by helping the patient to resist the urge to perform the behavior. By combining exposure with response prevention, the patient learns that the feared consequences do not take place, and anxiety decreases. Ultimately this leads to extinguishing the symptom. (For an excellent review of behavior therapy in children, see March et al. 1994). Bolton et al. (1983) used response prevention in 15 adolescents with OCD and achieved a "very good" response in 11. Often a combination of pharmacotherapy and behavioral therapy are used in children and adolescents.

▼ Adult Follow-Up Studies

Earlier Adult Studies

The early follow-up studies of adults with OCD are difficult to critically assess because of the lack of standardized diagnostic criteria and systematic ratings. For example, Ingram (1961) described a group of patients with obsessional states that included obsessive-compulsive neurosis, phobic-ruminative states, doubtfully schizophrenic, those with depressive features, and miscellaneous. There were no standardized diagnostic criteria at that time, so it is unclear which of those patients would have been diagnosed with OCD under current definitions. Additionally, there were few systematic rating scales for OCD severity or global functioning utilized in the studies, so it is difficult to make comparisons across studies at baseline and at follow-up. The severity of the patients' symptoms varied across reports, with different samplings of inpatients and outpatients. Interim treatments were limited to hospitalization, psychotherapy, electroconvulsive therapy (ECT), or leucotomy, and these are no longer the primary treatments of choice. Other methodological issues that limited their generalizability included the limited numbers of patients located at follow-up, the low percentage actually assessed in person at follow-up, and the lack of prospective design. The high frequency of comorbid diagnoses, which may be the primary or secondary diagnosis, complicated the interpretation of follow-up studies (Leonard et al. 1993) because it is problematic to assess how the comorbid diagnosis affects morbidity.

Follow-up studies on adults with OCD can be divided into those done before or after the availability of SRIs and the new behavioral therapy techniques. The early studies reported varied results, noting that anywhere from 29% to 61% of patients were unchanged or worse (Leonard et al. 1993). Specific descriptions from these early studies said that the patients were "cured," had "done quite well," had "experienced an episodic course with periods of severe illness," had "improved a little," were "no better," or were worse. Unfortunately, it was difficult to quantify how many patients were cured because of the different assessment approaches. For example, Kringlen (1965) found that at a 10-year follow-up of adults with obsessional neurosis, only 3 (3.3%) of 91 patients were cured, but 13 (14.3%) were "much improved," and 28 (30.8%) were "slightly improved" without specific quantification. Without systematic assessments and ratings it is difficult to draw conclusions about the outcome of adult OCD patients, other than to note that there was a wide range of severity.

There were seven reports (published in the English language) that could be considered the historical literature on the follow-up of OCD patients. Lewis (1936), in the earliest study, reported results generally consistent with later ones. Lewis reevaluated (in person) 50 patients at least 5 years after they were initially seen at the Maudsley Hospital. All but 2 had received interim treatment;

31 (62%) had been treated with psychotherapy combined with medicinal treatment, and 17 (34%) had been treated with intensive analytic psychotherapy either on an inpatient or outpatient basis. Lewis reported that 16 (32%) of the patients were quite well and had been so for years, 7 (14%) were much improved, 5 (10%) were quite well for years but then relapsed, 5 (10%) were a little improved, and 17 (34%) were no better or worse than when first seen.

Subsequent reports, although differing on specifics, also reported a mixed outcome. Pollitt (1957), used a questionnaire to reevaluate 101 of 150 (67%) patients with obsessional states and found that 61 (60%) of the patients reached a state of social adaptation, in which 31 (31%) were symptom-free. Interestingly, one patient (1%) had developed schizophrenia. Balslev-Olesen and Geert-Jorgensen (1959) found 19 of 52 (37%) patients were unchanged or worse after an unspecified follow-up period. Ingram (1961) found that 36 of 64 (56%) patients were unchanged or worse after a follow-up period of 5.9 (± 3.47) years, of whom 4 (6%) had developed schizophrenia. Kringlen (1965) reported that 27 of 91 (30%) patients were unchanged or worse after a 13- to 20-year follow-up period. Grimshaw (1965) reevaluated 100 (93.5%) patients 5.08 (± 3.43) years after a diagnosis of obsessional disorder had been made. Sixty-four percent were improved, 40% to the point of recovery or considerable improvement, which left 36% of the patients unchanged or worse. Lo (1967) reevaluated 88 Chinese patients who had been initially categorized into diagnostic groups much like those of Ingram's (obsessive-compulsive, phobic-ruminative, atypical obsessional) 3.9 (± 3.1) years after initial contact. Eleven (13%) were unchanged or worse, and 2 (2.3%) were schizophrenic.

The occasional report of a schizophrenia diagnosis having been assigned at follow-up raised the issue of whether OCD might turn into such a disorder. In four of these seven studies, 7 cases of schizophrenia and 6 cases of psychosis/borderline psychosis were reported from a total of 344 cases. Based on more recent follow-up studies, which do not support a continuity between the disorders, some schizophrenia patients were probably initially misdiagnosed as having OCD.

The only available treatments before the last decade were psychotherapy, ECT, and leucotomy. Three of these adult studies report the effect of leucotomy, which was once considered to be the treatment of choice for OCD. (The reader is referred to Chiocca and Martuza 1990 for a review of neurosurgical treatment of OCD.) Interestingly, leucotomy is occasionally recommended now for the truly severe and treatment-refractory patient, although the actual techniques have changed dramatically in recent years. Pollitt (1957) reported that half (15 of 31) of the cured group of patients had been leucotomized. Balslev-Olesen and Geert-Jorgensen (1959) reported that 8 of 10 (80%) lobotomized patients were improved, compared with 33 of 52 (63%) nonlobotomized patients. Finally, Ingram (1961) found that 10 of 18 (56%) leucotomized patients were improved at follow-up, versus 18 of 46 (40%) of nonleucotomized patients. These results would seem to indicate that leucotomy was sometimes effective, but without systematic comparison studies the conclusions are anecdotal.

Later Adult Studies

The more recent follow-up studies of adult OCD patients have involved either the current behavior therapy of choice, exposure with response prevention, or pharmacotherapy. Unfortunately, the literature has few systematic controlled behavioral treatment trials with prospective follow-up. Most studies do not report the number of patients actually screened, do not report specifics of concurrent pharmacotherapy, and do not have a comparison or control group. In one of their earliest reports, Marks et al. (1975) reevaluated 20 patients 2 years after treatment with in vivo exposure with self-imposed response prevention. They reported that 14 (70%) were much improved, 1 (5%) was improved, and 5 (25%) were "treatment failures." Nine patients required antidepressant therapy at some time during the follow-up phase, but specifics were not reported. It was not specified how the 20 subjects were chosen for follow-up from the 125 seen on the unit. It would have been interesting to know how the one-quarter of the 125 who refused behavioral treatment might have done at follow-up, but this was not the design.

Subsequently, Mawson et al. (1982) reported 2-year follow-up on 37 (92%) of 40 patients with OCD who had been randomly assigned to four double-blind conditions (15 hours in vivo exposure with either clomipramine or placebo; 30 hours in vivo exposure with either clomipramine or placebo). In the follow-up period, 7 of the 18 patients who had been originally assigned to the placebo group received (unspecified) tricyclics. The authors concluded that the sample as a whole was significantly improved on all measures, and that the more prolonged exposure treatment (30 vs. 15 sessions) predicted more improvement of rituals but not mood or social adjustment at follow-up. There was no drug effect on rituals at 2-year follow-up. Outcome was not predicted by initial anxiety or depression, sex, age, age at onset, or duration of rituals.

Foa and Goldstein (1978) reevaluated 19 of 21 patients who had been treated with continuous exposure to discomfort-evoking stimuli and prevention of discomfort-reducing rituals. After a mean follow-up period of 15 months (range: 3 months to 3 years), 12 (63%) patients had no symptoms, 4 (21%) were mildly to moderately symptomatic, and 3 patients (16%) had failed to respond to treatment.

Kasvikis and Marks (1988) followed up 39 of 49 patients 2 years after they had participated in a double-blind controlled study of exposure therapy and clomipramine treatment (clomipramine plus exposure compared with placebo plus exposure homework, therapist-accompanied exposure compared with self-exposure homework, and clomipramine plus exposure compared with clomipramine plus anti-exposure homework). At 2 years, there were no between-group differences; patients were significantly improved on all outcome measures compared with pretreatment. Seventy-one percent of patients had improved more than 25% on their target rituals (53% had more than 50% improvement) and 29% of patients had less than 25% improvement (actual N's not reported).

O'Sullivan et al. (1991) reevaluated 34 of 40 patients 6 years after treatment with exposure therapy (for 3 or 6 weeks) and with clomipramine or placebo (for 36 weeks). (It is of note that this was a self-selected sample because 110 had been screened but 46 did not meet inclusion criteria, 14 were suitable but refused treatment, and 10 dropped out of the study.) In the interim, 5 (15%) patients had received further exposure therapy and 24 (71%) had had pharmacotherapy. (Six patients had taken clomipramine, mean dose 100 mg/day.) At the time of follow-up, 20 (61%) patients were taking medication; 5 of those were on clomipramine, mean dose 85 mg/day (range 50–150 mg). The best predictor of long-term outcome was improvement at the end of initial treatment; better outcome was correlated with more exposure therapy (6 weeks vs. 3 weeks) and compliance with exposure therapy homework. The 5 patients on clomipramine at follow-up scored comparably on target rituals to the 13 drug-free patients and to the 15 patients on other medications. It is difficult to draw conclusions about the efficacy of clomipramine because low dosages were prescribed, and the subgroups contained small N's for comparisons. In summary, success with exposure therapy seemed to indicate better long-term outcome, and these results seem to be generally consistent with those of the early studies.

▼ Pediatric Follow-Up Studies

Early Pediatric Studies

Berman (1942) reported six cases of children with OCD and described their status at follow-up, which ranged from 6 months to 7 years. In one of the cases, the patient's "symptoms continued after discharge with frequent exacerbations and remissions" (p. 32). When seen 6 years later, "she was religiously preoccupied and felt as if she had sinned" (p. 32). Berman noted that this girl "developed trends suggestive of early schizophrenia" and raised the question as to "whether or not severe cases of obsessive-compulsive neurosis develop into schizophrenia" (p. 32). The case description is very typical for OCD and not suggestive of psychosis, yet the understanding of psychiatry was very different at that time. Berman wrote, "We cannot at present differentiate an obsessive-compulsive neurosis from a similar syndrome in a very early schizophrenia" (p. 33). Although the diagnostic criteria are different, his report speaks to the waxing and waning course of the illness and its chronicity. He concluded, "The prognosis is good for any one episode of neurosis," but "the long-term prognosis is much less favorable" (p. 38).

The earliest follow-up study of children and adolescents with OCD was reported by Warren (1960). Fifteen patients, ages 12–17 years, with "obsessive-compulsive conditions" (p. 816) were admitted to the hospital between 1949 and 1953 and were sought for reevaluation 5 years later. (These were the only patients admitted to the Maudsley Hospital with this as their primary diagnosis.) Onset of the disorder ranged from ages 4–10. There was no description of interim treatment, and the method of follow-up was unspecified (in-person or not). At follow-up, only 2 patients (13%) were completely recovered, although 4 patients (27%) continued to have only mild obsessions. The remaining 9 (60%) were categorized as being disabled from their illness. Specifically, 4 (27%) were somewhat disabled and 2 (13%) were severely disabled by their obsessional symptoms. Two (13%) were either in the hospital or required it, and 1 (7%) had been leucotomized. Warren noted that OCD "tends to continue or to recur" (p. 825) and raised the issue of the prognostic implications for these children when seen at an early stage.

Hollingsworth et al. (1980) reevaluated 10 of 17 (59%) patients with obsessive-compulsive neurosis who had met Judd's (1965) criteria 6.5 years (range: 1.5–14 years) earlier. The patients were sought after a retrospective review of 8,367 child and adolescent inpatient medical records, from which 50 cases were identified as having obsessive-compulsive neurosis, 17 of whom met Judd's criteria for OCD. Mean age at onset of OCD was 9.6 years (range: 3–15 years). Hollingsworth specifically noted psychopathology in an unusually large number (82%) of the parents. In the interim period between baseline and follow-up, all patients had received some form of psychotherapy. Ten percent of the patients also received (unspecified) behavior modification. Therapy lasted for an average of 17 months, typically on a once or twice weekly outpatient basis (three patients initially had inpatient treatment). No psychotropic drugs were administered except for one patient who was on imipramine for enuresis (no dosages or duration specified).

Hollingsworth et al. (1980) reported that, when evaluated at follow-up by structured interview, all 10 patients had improved, but only 3 (30%) had no obsessive thoughts or compulsions. Seven of the 10 patients (70%) reported that "obsessive-compulsive behavior still continued to some degree but was less than pretreatment level." Patients were doing well at school, but "all reported problems with their social life and peer relationships" and "only 3 of the 10 were dating" (p. 140). One of the 10 patients (10%) had "decompensated later [before follow-up] in an acute schizophrenic reaction which resolved without recurrence" (p. 140). Although these results compared favorably with other follow-up studies, Hollingsworth et al. concluded that "obsessive-compulsive neurosis in childhood is a disorder which seriously interferes with normal social and adaptive living and carries a poor long-term prognosis for complete resolution" (p. 144). Despite methodological issues about its retrospective design, low percentage of patients followed up (59%), lack of systematic rating scales, and lack of a control group, this study was an important early look at these children.

Later Pediatric Studies

The studies up until this point were done before the availability of the serotonin SRIs and the behavior therapy technique of exposure with response prevention. Bolton et al. (1983) reevaluated 14 of 15 patients (93%) who were at the Maudsley hospital between 1977 and 1981 (ages 12–18 at presentation) and who had participated in a treatment study of adolescents with primary OCD. This group represented the more severe end of the spectrum of OCD; 11 had been inpatients and 4 had been outpatients. Inpatient treatment was primarily self-imposed exposure with response prevention, but when children refused self-imposed discipline, the prevention was externally imposed by the hospital staff. The primary outpatient treatment was self-imposed response prevention with self-monitoring of symptoms; however, when this was not sufficient, an attempt was made to engage parents in response prevention. Clomipramine (of unspecified doses and duration) was administered to 5 patients: to 1 for obsessive-compulsive symptoms when it appeared other methods were unsuccessful, and to 4 other patients for anxiety and depression.

Bolton et al.'s (1983) follow-up was conducted 1.8 years (range:

9 months–4 years) later by interview with child and parents, either in person ($n = 8$; 57%) or by telephone ($n = 5$; 36%); 1 patient (7%) was currently in treatment, and 1 patient refused contact. Thirteen of the 15 patients (87%) improved after treatment. Seven patients (50%) appeared to be symptom free, 6 (43%) were mildly obsessional (less than 1 hour a day spent with symptoms), and 1 (7%) was severely incapacitated (between 1 and 4 hours a day spent with symptoms). Bolton et al. acknowledged that "these results apparently compare favorably with those of other treatment or follow-up studies of groups of obsessive compulsive adolescents" (p. 463), but without a control group it is difficult to make definitive conclusions. Subsequently, Bolton and colleagues have reevaluated 13 of the original 15 patients at 10-year follow-up and found that 7 had a chronic OCD course and 6 were symptom free (Derek Bolton, Ph.D., personal communication, July 2, 1993).

Allsopp and Verduyn (1988) retrospectively evaluated 20 of 26 subjects (77%)—identified by chart reviews as meeting Judd's (1965) criteria for OCD—who had initially been treated on an adolescent psychiatry unit between 1974 and 1979. Mean age of the subjects on first evaluation at the unit was 15 years (range: 12–18). Twenty-two patients had received some form of treatment before discharge from the unit, either on an inpatient ($n = 16$) or outpatient ($n = 6$) basis. Treatments included behavioral therapy with response prevention combined with family work ($n = 14$), as well as other therapeutic interventions (psychodynamic psychotherapy [$n = 1$], family therapy [$n = 2$], social skills therapy [$n = 1$], and pharmacotherapy using antidepressants, major tranquilizers, and ECT [$n = 1$] [all different patients]). Four patients received psychiatric treatment for problems other than OCD. An additional four subjects had received unspecified psychiatric treatment in the interim time. Follow-up, by means of a semistructured interview, took place an average of 9.8 years (range: 6.5–12 years) after discharge from the unit. At follow-up, 10 patients (50%) had a psychiatric disorder, and 10 (50%) were nonsymptomatic. Of the 10 symptomatic patients, 6 (30%) still had OCD, 2 (10%) had schizophrenia, and 2 (10%) had depression. The report did not specifically comment on whether those with diagnoses of schizophrenia at follow-up (retrospectively) appeared different at baseline from the other subjects. Baseline phenomenological variables did not distinguish the symptomatic and the asymptomatic group at follow-up. Interestingly, the patients who were free from symptoms at follow-up included all those whose symptoms had completely remitted during earlier contact. Although Allsopp and Verduyn's results appear favorable, the lack of complete follow-up data suggests a need for cautious interpretation.

In Denmark, Thomsen (in press) identified 61 children and adolescents with OCD who had been identified from case records of all pediatric patients ($N = 4,594$) previously admitted to the Children's Psychiatric Hospital from 1970 to 1986. Six people under the age of 18 were not sought for follow-up, and 47 of the remaining 55 subjects (85%) treated in childhood (30 inpatient, 31 outpatient) for OCD consented to an interview 6–22 years later (mean: 15.6). Initial treatments had included pharmacotherapy with SRIs ($n = 12$) and traditional antidepressants ($n = 3$), psychotherapy ($n = 47$), family therapy ($n = 32$), individual therapy ($n = 26$), and inpatient behavioral therapy ($n = 22$). At follow-up, 13 (28%) patients no longer had OCD symptoms. Ten patients (21%) had a phasic course with periods of often disabling OCD under stress, interrupted by long intervals (1 to several years) with mild or no obsessive-compulsive symptoms. Twelve patients (25.5%) had chronic OCD with constant, more or less disabling, OCD symptoms. Twelve patients (25.5%) had obsessive-compulsive symptoms (subclinical) not severe enough to meet criteria for OCD. Thomsen's report of a wide spectrum of severity at follow-up, ranging from one-quarter of the patients having a chronic disabling OCD to one-quarter with no OCD, suggested that the majority had some type of long-term obsessive-compulsive symptomatology.

Epidemiological Studies

Berg et al. (1989b) reevaluated 16 of 20 (80%) adolescents with OCD 2 years after having been initially identified from a large epidemiological study of 5,596 high school students in a county of New Jersey (Flament et al. 1988). As an epidemiological design, no interim treatment was specifically provided as a part of this study.

At follow-up, 5 patients (31%) still received a diagnosis of OCD, 4 (25%) were diagnosed with subclinical OCD, 2 (12%) with obsessive-compulsive personality (OCP), 5 (31%) with subclinical OCP, and 6 (37%) with other psychiatric disorders with obsessive-compulsive features. Only 2 patients (12%) received no diagnosis. (Percentages exceed 100% because personality disorder and other psychiatric disorders could be diagnosed in addition to OCD.) Co-morbid psychopathology and continued impaired functioning were also common in this group of patients with OCD. These data suggest that in these nonreferred cases of OCD, there was a varied outcome, with only a little over one-third who continued to meet the severity level for diagnostic criteria.

C. Z. Berg et al. (1989) wrote, "The most problematic area remains the diagnosis of OCP" (p. 533). One woman diagnosed with OCD at baseline was rated as subclinical OCP at follow-up because she found her perfectionistic behaviors useful in obtaining career goals. One wonders whether the woman adapted to her symptoms and no longer found them distressing. At the time of follow-up for the eight subjects diagnosed with OCP at baseline, only one still met criteria for this diagnosis at follow-up and two developed OCD. The authors wrote, "The diagnosis of OCP in adolescence as well as its relationship to OCD remains a major unsettled area" (p. 533).

NIMH Follow-Up Studies

The first systematic, controlled, prospective follow-up study of children and adolescents with OCD was conducted by Flament et al. (1990) with a group of 25 of 27 (93%) patients who had participated in a controlled clomipramine treatment study. The patients were systematically evaluated at baseline with structured interviews and rating scales and met DSM-III-R criteria for primary OCD. At baseline, the subjects ranged in age from 10–18 years old (mean: 14.4 years) and had had a mean age at onset of 4.1 years (range 1–10). Twenty-nine matched normal control subjects were also evaluated at baseline and follow-up.

After completion of the 5-week study, patients were referred to community practitioners for ongoing treatment, and all but two had received some form(s) of treatment (Flament et al. 1990). Although clomipramine was not commercially available at that time, seven patients received unspecified dosages of that medication for a duration that ranged from a few months to 3 years. Other pharmacotherapy treatments included other tricyclic antidepressants ($n = 5$), monoamine oxidase inhibitors ($n = 3$), neuroleptics ($n = 5$), anxiolytics ($n = 4$), and lithium ($n = 3$). Interim psychotherapies included individual psychotherapy ($n = 16$), group therapy ($n = 3$), family therapy ($n = 2$), residential treatment ($n = 3$), and hypnosis ($n = 1$).

At follow-up 2–7 years later (mean: 4.4), 17 (68%) patients still met criteria for OCD (mild [$n = 4$], moderate [$n = 9$], or severe [$n = 4$]). Of these 17 (68%) patients diagnosed with OCD, 12 (48%) also received additional current diagnoses for other psychiatric disorders. Of the 8 (32%) who did not have OCD at follow-up, 1 patient (4%) was diagnosed with atypical psychosis, and 7 patients (28%) did not receive any current psychiatric diagnosis and were considered completely well. At follow-up, 35% of the matched control group had a current psychiatric diagnosis, as compared with 72% of the patients. Diagnoses for the control group were most often drug and alcohol abuse, and there were no cases of OCD.

Flament et al. (1990) attempted to predict outcome based on baseline measures. The most striking finding was that an initial favorable response to clomipramine did not predict better long-term outcome, although the authors cautioned that treatment during the interim period was sparse and uncontrolled. (Neither clomipramine or other serotonin reuptake inhibitors were commercially available during the interim period.) Neither symptom severity, neurological impairment, nor family history of anxiety or depression predicted outcome. Flament et al. observed that "the most striking finding of this study is the continued psychopathology for this group of children" (p. 771), and thus corroborated earlier follow-up studies' findings of the chronicity of OCD.

Subsequently, in the largest prospective follow-up study of children and adolescents with OCD, Leonard et al. (1993) reported the outcome of 54 children and adolescents who had initially participated in treatment protocols for OCD. The study attempted to determine whether this group of patients who had had access to new psychopharmacological treatments would have improved long-term gains and whether there would be any predictors of outcome. Fifty-four children and adolescents were reevaluated 2–7 years (mean: 3.4 ± 1.0 years) after initial clomipramine treatment (Leonard et al. 1993). Information for 48 (89%) of the patients was from direct interview and for the remaining 6 (11%) from at least two sources. Interim treatments included medication ($n = 52$; 96%), behavioral therapy ($n = 18$; 33%), individual psychotherapy ($n = 29$; 54%), and family therapy ($n = 11$; 20%). Of the 18 subjects who received behavior therapy, only 10 received exposure with response prevention, and the other 8 had other behavioral techniques. (Of note, access to clomipramine maintenance became available to participants on an investigational basis in 1987, although the drug was not yet commercially available.) Twenty-six (48%) of the patients received long-term clomipramine maintenance from NIMH and participated in an 8-month double-blind desipramine substitution study to assess the need for continued drug treatment (Leonard et al. 1991).

Leonard et al. (1993) reported that at follow-up 23 subjects (43%) met diagnostic criteria for OCD. Ten subjects (18%) had subclinical OCD, 15 (28%) had features of OCD, and only 6 (11%) had no obsessions or compulsions. At least half of the patients in each OCD severity category were currently receiving medication. Only 3 (6%) of the 6 patients with no obsessive-compulsive symptoms were not receiving medication and might be considered in true remission. As a group, rating scales for OCD, anxiety, depression, and overall functioning were significantly improved over baseline. On the Yale-Brown Obsessive-Compulsive Scale, 80% of the patients were rated as "improved," 9% had "no change," and 9% were "worse."

Comorbid diagnoses were common at follow-up, and only two (4%) of the patients had no current comorbid diagnoses at follow-up (Leonard et al. 1993). Three patients developed psychotic disorders in the interim; one appeared to be a brief reactive psychosis while on medication; the others were a schizophreniform and a schizoaffective disorder. Ten patients required hospitalization in the interim. Interestingly, for the seven patients who were moderately to severely impaired at follow-up, the poor outcome was clinically judged to be due to a combination of the OCD, family dysfunction, and comorbid psychopathology. In a separate report, the findings about tic disorder at follow-up were detailed (Leonard et al. 1992). At follow-up, 59% ($n = 32$) had a lifetime history of tics, as compared with 57% ($n = 31$) at baseline. Eight patients (all male) met criteria for Tourette's syndrome (six had developed the disorder and two, it could be argued in retrospect, might have met criteria at baseline). The patients with Tourette's syndrome differed from other male patients only in having an earlier age at onset of OCD.

Leonard et al. (1993) reported that neither baseline OCD severity nor demographic variables predicted outcome at 2- to 7-year follow-up. A more severe OCD rating after an initial 5-week trial of clomipramine was associated with more severe OCD and poor functioning at follow-up. Additionally, a lifetime tic diagnosis at baseline and the presence of an Axis I disorder in a parent was associated with poorer outcome.

The patients in this later follow-up study (Leonard et al. 1993), which included more active interim treatment, appeared to do better than those reevaluated by Flament et al. (1990). One is tempted to infer that treatment interventions can improve long-term prognosis; however, without untreated control groups, one cannot conclude that the interventions were responsible. Obviously, the generalizability of these results to the general population is unknown because the more symptomatic patients may have been referred for the NIMH studies. Although some symptoms continued for the majority, in general the results were encouraging, with 81% of the subjects rated as improved at follow-up over baseline. Unfortunately, there was a small percentage of patients for whom OCD appeared to be chronic and unremitting, which was consistent with the early literature.

▼ Summary

Older follow-up studies of adults with OCD have generally reported continued morbidity, with 29%–61% of the patients unimproved. Similarly, follow-up studies of children and adolescents with OCD have noted a range of outcome, with a significant percentage of patients with continued difficulties and some who were severely handicapped.

With the new treatment interventions of the SRIs and exposure with response prevention behavior therapy, it was hoped that the long-term outcome might be improved for children and adolescents with OCD. The recent prospective follow-up study (Leonard et al. 1993), completed after new treatment interventions became available, reported that 81% of the subjects were improved at follow-up, although only 6% were in true remission. Seventy percent were taking medication specifically for OCD symptomatology at the time of follow-up. This would suggest that most children with OCD could expect significant improvement, but probably not remission, over time. Interestingly, baseline OCD severity did not predict long-term outcome, whereas short-term (5-week) drug response did. The study is consistent with early reports that there remained a small group of patients with significant difficulties despite treatment interventions. Further research is needed to determine whether treatment involving both exposure with response prevention behavior therapy and an SRI would offer long-term benefit over either done alone. Hopefully, as neurobiological research identifies the etiologies and risk factors for exacerbations, new treatment interventions will be developed and long-term outcome can be improved.

▼ References

Allsopp M, Verduyn C: A follow-up of adolescents with obsessive-compulsive disorder. Br J Psychiatry 154:829–834, 1988

American Psychiatric Association: Diagnostic and Statistical Manual of Mental Disorders, 3rd Edition, Revised. Washington, DC, American Psychiatric Association, 1987

Balslev-Olesen T, Geert-Jorgensen E: The prognosis of obsessive-compulsive neurosis. Acta Psychiatr Scand 136:232–241, 1959

Berg CJ, Rapoport JL, Wolff RP: Behavioral treatment for obsessive compulsive disorder in childhood, in Childhood Obsessive Compulsive Disorder. Edited by Rapoport JL. Washington, DC, American Psychiatric Association, 1989, pp 169–185

Berg CZ, Rapoport JL, Whitaker A, et al: Childhood obsessive com-
    pulsive disorder: a two-year prospective follow-up of a commu-
    nity sample. J Am Acad Child Adolesc Psychiatry 28:528–533,
    1989

Berman L: Obsessive-compulsive neurosis in children. J Nerv Ment
    Dis 95:26–39, 1942

Bolton D, Collins S, Steinberg D: The treatment of obsessive-com-
    pulsive disorder in adolescence: a report of fifteen cases. Br J
    Psychiatry 142:456–464, 1983

Chiocca EA, Martuza RL: Neurosurgical therapy of obsessive-com-
    pulsive disorder, in Obsessive-Compulsive Disorders: Theory and
    Management. Edited by Jenike MA, Baer L, Minichiello WE.
    Chicago, IL, Year Book Medical Publishers, 1990, pp 283–294

Despert L: Differential diagnosis between obsessive-compulsive neu-
    rosis and schizophrenia in children, in Psychopathology of Child-
    hood. New York, Grune & Stratton, 1955

DeVeaugh-Geiss J, Moroz G, Biederman J et al: Clomipramine hy-
    drochloride in childhood and adolescent obsessive-compulsive
    disorder—a multicenter trial. J Am Acad Child Adolesc Psychia-
    try 31:45–49,1992

Flament M, Rapoport JL, Berg CJ, et al: Clomipramine treatment of
    childhood obsessive compulsive disorder: a double-blind con-
    trolled study. Arch Gen Psychiatry 42:977–983, 1985

Flament M, Whitaker A, Rapoport J, et al: Obsessive compulsive dis-
    order in adolescence: an epidemiological study. J Am Acad Child
    Adolesc Psychiatry 27:764–771, 1988

Flament MF, Koby E, Rapoport JL, et al: Childhood obsessive-com-
    pulsive disorder: a prospective follow-up study. J Child Psychol
    Psychiatry 31:363–380, 1990

Foa EB, Goldstein A: Continuous exposure and complete response
    prevention of obsessive-compulsive neurosis. Behavior Therapy
    9:821–829, 1978

Freud S: Notes on a case of obsessional neurosis (1909), in The
    Standard Edition of the Complete Psychological Works of Sig-
    mund Freud, Vol. 10. Edited by Strachey J. London, England,
    Hogarth Press, 1955, Vol 10, pp 153–318

Goodman WK, McDougle CJ, Price LH, et al: Beyond the serotonin hypothesis: a role for dopamine in some forms of obsessive compulsive disorder? J Clin Psychiatry 51(suppl):36–43, 1990

Grimshaw L: The outcome of obsessional disorder: a follow-up study of 100 cases. Br J Psychiatry 111:1051–1056, 1965

Hollingsworth CE, Tanguay PE, Grossman L, et al: Long-term outcome of obsessive-compulsive disorder in childhood. J Am Acad Child Psychiatry 19:134–144, 1980

Insel TR: Toward a neuroanatomy of obsessive-compulsive disorder. Arch Gen Psychiatry 49:739–744, 1992

Insel TR, Mueller EA, Alterman I, et al: Obsessive compulsive disorder and serotonin: is there a connection? Biol Psychiatry 20: 1174–1188, 1985

Ingram IM: Obsessional illness in mental hospital patients. Journal of Mental Science 107:382–402, 1961

Janet P: Les Obsessions et la Psychiatrie, Vol. 1. Paris, France, Felix Alan, 1903

Jenike MA: Pharmacologic treatment of obsessive compulsive disorders. Psychiatr Clin North Am 15:895–919, 1992

Judd LJ: Obsessive compulsive neurosis in children. Arch Gen Psychiatry 12:136–143, 1965

Kanner L: Child Psychiatry, 3rd Edition. Springfield, IL, Charles C. Thomas, 1962

Kasvikis Y, Marks IM: Clomipramine, self-exposure and therapist accompanied exposure in OCD: two-year follow-up. Journal of Anxiety Disorders 2:291–298, 1988

Kringlen E: Obsessional neurotics: a long-term follow-up. Br J Psychiatry 111:709–722, 1965

Lenane MC, Swedo SE, Leonard HL, et al: Psychiatric disorders in first degree relatives of children and adolescents with obsessive compulsive disorder. J Am Acad Child Adolesc Psychiatry 29:407–412, 1990

Leonard HL, Swedo SE, Rapoport JL, et al: Treatment of childhood obsessive compulsive disorder with clomipramine and desipramine: a double-blind crossover comparison. Arch Gen Psychiatry 46:1088–1092, 1989

Leonard HL, Swedo SE, Lenane MC, et al: A double-blind desipramine substitution during long-term clomipramine treatment in children and adolescents with obsessive compulsive disorder. Arch Gen Psychiatry 48:922–927, 1991

Leonard HL, Swedo SE, Rapoport JL: The diagnosis of Tourette's syndrome at two to seven year follow-up of 54 obsessive-compulsive children. Am J Psychiatry 149:1244–1251, 1992

Leonard HL, Swedo SE, Lenane MC, et al: A 2- to 7-year follow-up study of 54 obsessive-compulsive children and adolescents. Arch Gen Psychiatry 50:429–439, 1993

Lewis A: Problems of obsessional illness. Proceedings of the Royal Society of Medicine 29:325–336, 1936

Lo WH: A follow-up study of obsessional neurotics in Hong-Kong Chinese. Br J Psychiatry 113:823–832, 1967

March JS, Mulle K, Herbel B: Behavioral psychotherapy for children and adolescents with obsessive compulsive disorder: an open trial of a new protocol driven treatment package. J Am Acad Child Adolesc Psychiatry 33:333–341, 1994

Marks IM: Fears, Phobias, and Rituals: Anxiety and Their Disorders. Oxford, England, Oxford University Press, 1987

Marks IM, Hodgson R, Rachman S: Treatment of chronic obsessive-compulsive disorder by in vivo exposure: a two year follow-up and issues in treatment. Br J Psychiatry 127:349–364, 1975

Mawson D, Marks IM, Ramm L: Clomipramine and exposure for chronic obsessive compulsive rituals: two year follow-up and further findings. Br J Psychiatry 140:11–18, 1982

O'Sullivan G, Noshirvani J, Marks I, et al: Six-year follow-up after exposure and clomipramine therapy for obsessive compulsive disorder. J Clin Psychiatry 52:150–155, 1991

Pauls DL, Towbin KE, Leckman JF, et al: Gilles de la Tourette's syndrome and obsessive compulsive disorder: evidence supporting a genetic relationship. Arch Gen Psychiatry 43:1180–1182, 1986

Pollitt J: Natural history of obsessional states: a study of 150 cases. BMJ 26:194–198, 1957

Rettew DC, Swedo SE, Leonard HL, et al: Obsessions and compulsions across time in 79 children and adolescents with obsessive compulsive disorder. J Am Acad Child Adolesc Psychiatry 31:1050–1056, 1992

Riddle MA, Scahill L, King RA, et al: Double-blind, crossover trial of fluoxetine and placebo in children and adolescents with obsessive compulsive disorder. J Am Acad Child Adolesc Psychiatry 31:1062–1069, 1992

Rutter M, Tizard J, Whitmore K: Education, Health and Behavior. London, England, Longmans, 1970

Suess L, Halpern MS: Obsessive-compulsive disorder: the religious perspective, in Obsessive Compulsive Disorder in Children and Adolescents. Edited by Rapoport JL. Washington, DC, American Psychiatric Press, 1989, pp 311–325

Swedo SE, Rapoport JL: Neurochemical and neuroendocrine considerations of obsessive compulsive disorders in childhood, in Application of Basic Neuroscience to Child Psychiatry. Edited by Deutsch SI, Weizman A, Weizman R. New York, Plenum, 1990, pp 275–284

Swedo SE, Rapoport JL, Leonard HL, et al: Obsessive compulsive disorder in children and adolescents: clinical phenomenology of 70 consecutive cases. Arch Gen Psychiatry 46:335–341, 1989

Thomsen PH: Obsessive compulsive disorder in Danish children and adolescents: a follow-up study. European Child and Adolescent Psychiatry, in press

Thomsen PH, Mikkelsen HU: Children and adolescents with obsessive-compulsive disorder: the demographic and diagnostic characteristics of 61 Danish patients. Acta Psychiatr Scand 83: 262–266, 1991

Warren W: Some relationships between the psychiatry of children and of adults. Journal of Mental Science 106:815–826, 1960

World Health Organization: The ICD-10 Classification of Mental and Behavioral Disorders, Clinical Descriptions and Diagnostic Guidelines. Geneva, Switzerland, World Health Organization, 1992

Chapter 9

Pervasive Developmental, Psychotic, and Allied Disorders

John Scott Werry, M.D.

Included here are a variety of disorders, all of which are characterized by bizarre, eccentric, or extremely unusual behavior ranging from the pervasive developmental disorders and psychoses such as schizophrenia, through to schizotypal and schizoid disorders. With the exception of autism, few of these disorders have attracted much systematic study of their occurrence and features in children and adolescents, let alone their long-term outcome. Much of what follows is necessarily sparse and aimed primarily at attracting attention to the need for research, especially because, in addition to causing considerable chronic disability, many of these disorders are probably similar to or precursors of their adult counterparts. Study of their origins in childhood should therefore have important implications for prevention or mitigation of the considerable disability to patients, grief to their families, and cost to the nation that they cause.

Terminology and diagnostic criteria used will generally be the DSM-IV criteria (American Psychiatric Association 1994). ICD-10 (World Health Organization 1992) is also referred to. Because there has been close cooperation, especially in the child and adolescent area, there is now less difference between DSM and ICD in the disorders to be discussed here (see Rutter and Schopler 1992).

▼ Autism, Asperger's Syndrome, and Pervasive Developmental Disorder Not Otherwise Specified

General Issues

Autism is characterized by severe delays or impairments in social interaction, in relationships (primarily deficits), and in communication (language, gesture, play); it is also characterized by restricted repetitive and stereotyped patterns of behavior, interests, and activities. All have their onset before age 3.

Asperger's syndrome, new to DSM-IV (American Psychiatric Association 1994), differs only in that language and cognitive development are normal. Asperger's syndrome is, therefore, in many cases, phenotypically at least, a mild version of autism (see Rutter and Schopler 1992). DSM-IV/ICD-10 definitions are narrower than Asperger's own (see Wolff 1991b) and others (e.g., Petti and Vela 1990; Tantam 1988a), which had blurred the boundaries with schizotypal disorders. Its sudden rise in popularity scarcely reflects the state of knowledge about it and it should be regarded as an interesting category awaiting validation (Szatmari 1992).

Pervasive development disorder, not otherwise specified (PDD-NOS) is used when the disorder has its onset after age 3 or when not quite all the criteria for autism are met. There is some controversy as to whether these three disorders are distinctive or merely variants of an autistic spectrum (Szatmari 1992). The data on outcome do not permit differentiation at this time so they will be treated here as variants.

Most of the diagnostic criteria in DSM-IV are only elaborations of Kanner's (1943) original criteria for autism, but the road to DSM-IV has not been smooth and the existence of these original criteria complicates greatly the question of long-term outcome, because such studies were of necessity begun or completed before DSM-IV. These studies present seven major problems:

1. The promiscuity in diagnosis, deplored by Kanner (1971a), which is likely to make outcome appear somewhat better than it really is.
2. The lumping together of all psychoses under childhood schizophrenia from about 1960 through to 1980. This is illustrated in one of the longest follow-up studies of psychotic children (Howells and Guirguis 1984). However, most psychoses are rare before about age 12 and with a few exceptions (e.g., PDD and the rare disintegrative disorder) do not begin until age 6 or 7 (Werry 1992). It is, therefore, sometimes possible to dissect samples into probably PDD and probably schizophrenic.
3. Autism is not an all or nothing disorder (Lotter 1974; Rutter and Schopler 1988); it varies in severity. There is therefore a problem of boundaries. Where to draw the line has been a discretionary issue, and variability across clinicians and studies is to be expected.
4. The studies reveal associated severe brain damage. Knobloch and Pasamanick (1975) and Wing and Gould (1979) have shown that damaged infants and children exhibit autistic features and that the more severe the damage, the greater the likelihood such features will be present. Though this has not been an exclusionary criterion in DSM, the tacit consensus in the past seems to have been that the diagnosis should not be made when the child is profoundly and generally retarded developmentally, and when there is clear evidence of neurological or physical disability. Further, this group seems to cluster separately from autism on multivariate analyses (Szatmari 1992).
5. There is a problem of biased sampling. As Gillberg (1991) points out, most studies have reported on clinic-referred cases, which are biased toward greater severity and worse outcome. The few studies into adulthood have sometimes relied on obtaining volun-

teers through newspaper advertisements (e.g., Rumsey et al. 1985—this study also contained some of Kanner's original cases). There has also been a tendency to exclude certain mostly poor prognostic cases, most conspicuously those that develop seizures or other medical complications or that were untestable (e.g., Rumsey et al. 1985; Szatmari et al. 1989).

6. The rate of improvement is uneven. There is some evidence (Rutter 1985a; Wing 1989) that loss of some autistic features may occur more rapidly in later adolescence or beyond, although the evidence is not unanimous (Kobayashi et al. 1992). Although the number of subjects collectively in studies is large (in excess of 500), the majority are adolescents, not adults. This may cause overestimation of disability at outcome.

7. There is a lack of formal studies and specific measures. Most details of adult status are global, vague, and anecdotal, not factual and quantitative.

Summary of Outcome Studies

In contrast to most of the other disorders here, there is a relatively large number of total subjects (>500) and reviews (DeMyer et al. 1981; Gillberg 1991; Lotter 1974; Mesibov 1983; Prior and Werry 1986; Rutter 1985a; Werry 1979; Wing 1989), all of which use much the same data and come to rather similar conclusions. Thus, it is unnecessary to review individual studies except those that are new or of particular interest. Although most of the studies are subject to the errors noted above, data are consistent and allow reasonable extrapolation to address long-term outcome.

There are three distinct patterns of social outcome. In the first pattern, most individuals (90%) remain socially and intellectually handicapped and unable to look after themselves fully. However, the range of disability varies from severely (two-thirds) to moderately (one-quarter) handicapped (Wing 1989). In all this, there is a resemblance to mentally retarded persons; the needs and type of care provided are usually similar. In the past (e.g., DeMyer et al. 1981), institutional care was common, but current trends have changed this (Mesibov 1983) (e.g., in Australia [Prior and Werry

1986] and in Japan [Kobayashi et al. 1992]). In spite of continuing significant handicap, most individuals show a considerable slow degree of improvement in their more severe autisticlike features (Mesibov 1983; Wing 1989), especially improvements in hyperactivity, stereotyped behavior, aloofness, or unrelatedness. Nevertheless, conspicuous oddity (Rutter 1985a) and disturbed behaviors such as aggression (Wing 1989) may remain. Thus, at adulthood, most (at least half) have insufficient criteria to merit the DSM diagnosis of autism except as a residual state (Gillberg 1991; Rumsey et al. 1985). At least half (Mesibov 1983) acquire some degree of language, although usually limited and with syntactical, pronominal, or pragmatic abnormalities (Rutter 1985a).

A second pattern of social outcome is that a small number of affected individuals improve dramatically. About 10% are able to receive normal education and appear to function as independent adults (Wing 1989). However, even these individuals retain some autistic features discernible to the experienced eye—described as literality, rigidity, impaired ability to read social signals, stilted language, lack of empathy, and social awkwardness (Kanner 1971a; Rutter 1985a; Wing 1989). Rumsey et al. (1985) noted, in addition, a marked discrepancy between IQ and social function (lower); they also noted anxiety, obsessive-compulsive traits, and stereotypes. Gillberg and Steffenburg (1987) noted conspicuous "oddness." Kobayashi et al. (1992) found that none of those employed were in service (that is, person-to-person) industries.

The last pattern of social outcome is that a small number of impaired individuals deteriorate. Although in some cases the deterioration is the result of institutionalization, in other cases there is no apparent cause (Rutter 1985a). Gillberg and Steffenburg (1987) noted this aggression, reactivation of autistic core symptoms, and/or deterioration in language in over half their cases around puberty. In many, this deterioration lasted for less than 2 years, although Kobayashi et al. (1992) found it to be somewhat more prolonged.

Some impaired individuals develop medical complications. The size of this group is unclear, although seizures (not necessarily with deterioration) are a frequent, sometimes late (that is, in adolescence) complication with a possible occurrence as high as 20%–30% (Gillberg 1991; Kobayashi et al. 1992; Rutter 1985a). There is prob-

ably an increase in mortality accounted for by some of the neurological disorders (e.g., tuberous sclerosis) associated with autism
(Gillberg 1991; Kobayashi et al. 1992).

Sometimes, other psychiatric disorders appear. The one of greatest interest is schizophrenia because, as noted, at one stage autism
was classified within the general category of childhood schizophrenia (see Prior and Werry 1986; Volkmar and Cohen 1991). There are
now a few studies (see Szatmari et al. 1989; Volkmar and Cohen
1991; Wolff et al. 1991) that show that children diagnosed as having
autism may later develop schizophrenia, although this is a rare event
(0.6%), and the risk is no higher than the risk in the population as
a whole. The exception is the study by Howells and Guirguis (1984)
in which, as deduced from the age at onset (3 years or under), the
majority of subjects (13 or 14 out of 20) probably had pervasive
developmental disorders. They found that most of the subjects
could be diagnosed as having schizophrenia using Feigner but not
Schneiderian criteria. However, as Rumsey et al. (1985) point out,
there is good reason to suspect this diagnosis because the typical
clinical state was a deficit one commonly described as outcome in
autism; positive schizophrenic symptoms were only suspected from
patient behavior, not reported by the subjects, and were much more
common in the late-onset group most likely to have had schizophrenia, not PDD; and there were no positive family histories of schizophrenia. Also, as Gillberg (1991) points out, because of their
behavior, many of her subjects have been misdiagnosed as schizophrenic after they passed from the child to the adult service. In a
long-term follow-up by Weber (cited in Wolff 1991a, 1991b), of
400 cases originally diagnosed by Asperger as having his syndrome,
only two cases had developed schizophrenia.

Wing (1989) states that hypersensitivity and affective disorders
are common but this is not based on formal study. Rumsey et al.
(1985) found that none of their adult sample warranted any further
diagnoses than autism or residual autism. None had hallucinations
or delusions or formal thought disorder, although two patients did
report rather bizarre but temporary delusional beliefs during childhood. The authors did note that if the history of autism was not
known, subjects may have been misdiagnosed as having anxiety disorders, or schizoid or compulsive personality disorders. In the

absence of further data, then, it seems safest to say that the development of other psychiatric disorders (as opposed to symptoms) in autism is unusual, but that much more research is needed.

Treatment and Outcome

Because of its severity, autism is unlikely to be untreated. Further, the number and types of treatment used over the years are bewildering, and subject to fads and fashions (see Gillberg 1989). This in itself suggests that treatment is without dramatic effect, although there have been a few efforts to evaluate treatment systematically. Rutter (1985b) suggests that no treatment can override the basic handicap, that treatment is most effective against nonspecific and not core problems, such as language and intelligence, that it seems to be situation specific, and that structured behavioral and educational approaches that take place in both home and school are best. All these data relate to relatively short-term outcomes.

There are no good data by which to evaluate whether treatment can influence long-term outcome, although it is fairly clear that any effects are modest (Gillberg 1991; Rutter 1985a, 1985b). The fact that cases that do very well have all been treated probably reflects selection bias (for treatment) rather than the effect of treatment because there are no adequate controlled studies (Gillberg 1991). The best that can be said is that it seems reasonable to assume that treatment that follows the principles set out by Rutter (1985b) is likely to produce a better adapted adult. These principles include the goal to foster normal development; thus, they involve a focus on intellectual, linguistic, and social development, as well as reduction of rigidity and stereotyping, the elimination of nonspecific, maladaptive behaviors, and the alleviation of family distress. In each of these areas, the approach needs to be individualized, direct, structured, and developmentally appropriate for the particular child. Availability of this treatment will vary with parental income and where the person lives. Nevertheless, it is also clear that even the best treatment cannot cure autism and that considerable disability remains.

Other Factors Affecting Outcome

There is rather better data here than on treatment. The variable
most clearly affecting outcome is severity of the disorder, however
measured. The two most robust indicators of severity are IQ and
language development (DeMyer et al. 1981; Gillberg 1991; Kobayashi et al. 1992; Lotter 1974; Prior and Werry 1986; Rutter
1985a) or equivalents such as severity of the disorder (DeMyer et
al. 1981; Wing 1989). An IQ of less than 50 and/or lack of communicative speech at age 5 foreshadow severe handicap through life
(Gillberg 1991; Rutter 1985a), although among those without
these criteria, the prognosis for a good outcome is said to be still
only 50% (Rutter 1985a). IQ and language scores parallel each
other and have been shown to be fairly stable in autistic children
(Campbell and Green 1985; Freeman et al. 1985), although relationships to scores in adulthood have not been investigated. The
powerful prognostic effect of IQ and language suggest that most
good outcome cases may well lie in the Asperger's category (Gillberg 1991).

The only other risk factor of any importance is a diagnosed physical disorder, some of which—such as tuberose sclerosis—will determine the ultimate prognosis. Seizures are said to increase the risk
of deterioration (Gillberg 1991). Fragile X may also influence prognosis (see Gillberg 1991).

Current Work on Treatment and Outcome

The standard of research in child psychopathology has increased
enormously in the last decade or so, and there are now several centers with a special interest in autism and well-studied large samples.
There are, however, no really promising leads on treatment or etiology that offer prospects of a breakthrough to radically alter outcome in PDD. What is most likely to happen is much better
documentation of what happens in adulthood and through multivariate and meta-analytic techniques and assessment of the effect
of existing treatment programs. Most treatment programs, apart
from whatever is faddish (currently, facilitated communication),
seem to be qualitatively similar at the core, differing only in inten-

sity, comprehensiveness across environments, and the degree to which they are behavioral/educational/problem oriented, and/or bound by the shibboleths of the past such as psychodynamic theory or parent-blaming.

Summary

Autism is a disorder that varies in severity, but clinically diagnosed autism has a disastrous effect on development. The best prognostic indicators are IQ and language development at age 5 or 6. Few diagnosed cases will ever achieve anything approaching normality, and even those that do remain discernibly different in their odd behavior, concrete thinking, and impaired social intelligence. The prognostic indicators suggest that most good outcome cases would now receive a diagnosis of Asperger's syndrome. Although the majority of clinical cases of PDD will remain seriously handicapped as adults, most will improve slowly, especially in their ability to relate and in the loss of the more conspicuous aspects of the disorder. At least half will achieve some degree of usable language, although mostly stilted and limited. A small group will show deterioration at adolescence, and a few will die.

The most prominent feature of the disorder in adulthood is a residual state characterized by rigidity and by impaired motivation, language, empathy, and interpersonal and other social behaviors. Apart from the unequivocal fact that no treatment is curative, the long-term impact of treatment is unclear. It seems reasonable to assume from short-term studies and from other seriously handicapping disorders that the adult deficit state will be influenced to some degree by the amount and continuity of social and educational/occupational stimulation that the subject has had, and continues to get. Epilepsy will develop in a significant minority, sometimes at adolescence. This merely reflects the fact that autism is a brain disorder, or, more properly, a group of brain disorders of very early onset, a few of which are known but the vast majority of which remain to be elucidated. Asperger's syndrome requires validation as to its separateness from autism but its prognosis should be much better, simply because it starts from a much better level of function, suggesting either milder or a different type of brain dysfunction. However, Asperger's syndrome may have just as close a relationship with schizoid personality disorder as with autism (Szatmari 1992; see also below).

▼ Other Pervasive Developmental Disorders

Childhood Disintegrative Disorder

This ICD-9/10 and DSM-IV disorder is characterized by healthy development for at least the first 2 years of life followed by loss of at least two previously acquired skills (language, social, bowel/bladder, motor, play). Kanner (1971a) refers to this as Heller's disease. Volkmar (1992) points out that there are two competing views— one that it is an encephalopathy and the other that it is a late-onset autism. This in turn reflects the fact that some cases have been associated with a variety of neurological disorders, but most have not. Volkmar's (1992) review found 77 reported cases. The mean age at onset was 3.3 years and the sex ratio was four males to one female. The clinical symptoms are similar to autism. There is a recent report of five more cases (Malhotra and Singh 1993), most with an age at onset of 4 years.

Follow-up has been limited in both number and duration (Volkmar 1992), but there are two outcomes. The least frequent outcome and not surprisingly the outcome that is most identified with neurodegenerative disorders is continued progression; however, the majority of cases arrest (Malhotra and Singh 1993; Volkmar 1992; Werry 1979). Although it is not possible to state at this stage what the definitive outcome in adulthood will be, apart from the small percentage who continue to deteriorate and/or die, the course in childhood and adolescence suggests that adult outcome is similar to that for autism—most cases are severely to moderately disabled intellectually and socially, and there are no reported cases of complete recovery. It is hoped that the inclusion of this disorder in both DSM-IV and ICD-10 will lead to better recognition and better long-term outcome studies, although there seems little doubt that the disability is lifelong.

Rett's Disorder

This new DSM-IV/ICD-10 disorder is of only recent recognition, and many cases in the past are presumed to have been misdiagnosed as autism. The characteristic features are healthy development until at least the first 5–6 months; between 5 and 48 months there is deceleration of head circumference, loss of acquired purposeful hand movements, appearance of characteristic stereotyped hand movements, loss of social engagement, poor coordination, and delay or impairment of language development. Although the disorder may at first resemble autism in severe social withdrawal, this is said to gradually improve later. Cases followed into adulthood show an extremely poor outcome—much worse than autism and including marked motor impairment not seen in autism (Tsai 1992). Again, developing and widespread pediatric recognition of this disorder and its inclusion in official psychiatric taxonomies should lead to better research on long-term outcome, which will define more precisely what improves (e.g., social reactivity) and what probably does not (intellectual and motor status).

▼ Schizophrenia

Introduction

Andreasen and Carpenter (1993) describe the disorder thus:

> Schizophrenia is a leading public health problem. The life time prevalence is high (0.5–1.0%, depending on the definition), morbidity is severe, and mortality is significant. Schizophrenia often begins relatively early in life, frequently leads to social and economic impairment, and typically leaves traces on its victims for the remainder of their lives. Schizophrenia results in great suffering for both patients and their families. Its cost to society is also great, exceeding the financial burden of cancer . . ." (p. 200)

They go on to discuss at some length the evolution of the concept and diagnosis of the disorder from Kraepelin and Bleuler to DSM-IV. Briefly stated, this was first slowly away from Kraepelin's rather narrow and prognostically ominous dementia praecox pervading all aspects of cognitive and behavioral function, to a period of elasticity (in North America) in which psychosis was seen as a matter of severity rather than of qualitative specific symptomatology. Beginning in the 1970s, there was a countermove to narrow, specify, operationalize, and ultimately internationalize the criteria. This countermove culminated first in DSM-III (American Psychiatric Association 1980), then in DSM-III-R (American Psychiatric Association 1987), and now in DSM-IV and ICD-10 (see Andreasen and Carpenter 1993; Andreasen and Flaum 1991).

Variation in diagnostic criteria is obviously important in any review of long-term outcome because today's subjects were diagnosed by yesterday's criteria. Nevertheless, the central core of schizophrenia in DSM-III and DSM-IV is much the same as it always was: positive symptoms of delusions, hallucinations, disorganized speech and thought, disorganized or catatonic behavior, and negative symptoms of affective flattening, alogia, avolition, all with marked interference with social and occupational/educational function. What has changed is the precision of description of the core symptoms and, in DSM, the requirement of a 6-month duration. Despite all this, Andreasen and Carpenter (1993) emphasize that schizophrenia is diverse in symptomatology and probably in etiologies, which, despite some attractive theories, remain unknown.

Early-Onset Schizophrenia

There have been a number of reviews of the history of the study of schizophrenia in children (Beitchman 1985; Eisenberg 1957; Kanner 1971a; Werry 1979). Up to about 1960, the criteria were much the same as in adults, with Kanner separating out autism in 1943. After 1960, under the influence of the "psychosis as severity" concept in both North America and the United Kingdom, two things occurred. The first was an extension of the diagnosis of childhood psychosis to include any major deviation in development other than mental retardation, and the second was a lumping together under a single DSM-II (American Psychiatric Association 1968) and ICD-8 (World Health Organization 1968) rubric called "childhood schizophrenia." Soon there was a major revolt against this led by Kolvin (1971) and Rutter (1972), and in 1980, in DSM-III, early-onset schizophrenia (EOS) was again separated from other childhood psychoses and, as before, was considered part of and the same disorder as in adults.

Schizophrenia has not been reported reliably in children under the age of 4–5 (Werry 1992) and is rare until adolescence, when frequency begins to rise quickly to reach a peak in the decade 15–24 in males and about 5 years later in females. Recent studies suggest that females may have a lower lifetime risk and a milder course (Iacono and Beiser 1992). Most studies of child and/or adolescent schizophrenia are of clinic cases, and there seem to be no epidemiological studies of children under age 15. Figures from one study of a total birth cohort of 11,093 in Goteborg, Sweden (Gillberg et al. 1986) showed an incidence of about 0.25% between the ages of 13 and 19 years admitted to hospital; however, only a quarter (0.06%) of these admissions occurred for subjects under the age of 15. As in most other studies (see Werry 1992), boys outnumbered girls by two to one. Although these figures are subject to local variation and errors from small numbers, they fit reasonably well with overall lifetime-risk figures and ages of maximum risk. Most cases had been seen first in adult services.

Methodological Problems in Outcome Studies

Diagnosis. Variations just described mean that there have been three distinct phases of research—pre-1960 and DSM-II, pre-1980 and DSM-III, and post–DSM-III. The first period (see Eisenberg 1957) is difficult to evaluate because most studies included cases that today would not be considered schizophrenia. The middle period is misleading in that most of the studies of "childhood schizophrenia" are actually of autism, and even those that might be of schizophrenia are difficult to interpret because of vague and all-encompassing criteria. Nevertheless, reviews (Beitchman 1985; Werry 1992) have been able to apply acceptable DSM-III or later diagnostic criteria to a small group of studies, sufficient to indicate what the outcome in EOS might be.

Limited number and acceptability of studies. Until very recently, the study of early-onset schizophrenia seems to have been eclipsed by other disorders, so that there have been few studies, and the number is further reduced by those studies that have overly broad diagnostic criteria, have severe methodological problems, or that are otherwise uninterpretable (see Werry 1992). Even fewer addressed long-term outcome. None can be considered entirely methodologically satisfactory by today's standards of research in adult schizophrenia, especially in use of similarly selected patient control groups, prospective design, measures of established reliability and validity at all stages, adequate record of treatment, and so on.

Subject selection and attrition. Older studies reviewed by Eisenberg (1957) are almost certainly biased toward severity (institutionalized), and subjects were not treated with antipsychotic drugs, which makes outcome look worse than it probably is. Later studies (e.g., Gillberg et al. 1993; Schmidt 1995; Werry et al. 1991) have made some attempt to look at the issue of sampling, and in general they seem somewhat more representative, although most subjects are still selected by inpatient admission. Subject attrition is not serious except in M. H. Schmidt (personal communication, 1995).

Age at onset. Childhood-onset (usually inappropriately called prepubertal) schizophrenic psychosis is rare and, not surprisingly therefore, with one exception (Eggers 1978, 1989) the studies concern mostly adolescent-onset subjects. This means little that is definitive can be said about childhood-onset schizophrenia, although there are some indicators. It may be noted that research increasingly suggests that often the schizophrenic process begins well before the onset of psychosis, even congenitally (see DeLisi 1992; Murray et al. 1992); so that current grouping of child-, adolescent- and adult-onset schizophrenia based on appearance of psychosis may be misleading. There are important implications in this for the relationship of schizophrenia and its precursor states to child psychiatry.

Retrospectiveness. All studies are retrospective and based on chart reviews as to initial diagnosis, symptoms, and predictors. This means that studies contain unknown errors of sampling, diagnosis, and measurement.

Initial misdiagnosis. An initial diagnosis of schizophrenia not infrequently may differ from later diagnoses, especially bipolar mood disorder and/or schizoaffective disorder (see Carlson 1990; Eggers 1989; Werry et al. 1991), but also other diagnoses (McClellan et al. 1993). Most of these misdiagnosed cases, if undetected, will influence outcome favorably. There is also reason to believe that some, and possibly the first, episodes of schizophrenia attract another psychotic diagnosis (NOS, brief reactive, drug induced) (McClellan et al. 1993). Some cases diagnosed as schizophrenia are some kind of brief psychosis in adolescents with personality disorders (Kafantaris et al. 1993; McClellan et al. 1993).

Summary of Long-Term Outcome Studies

Eisenberg (1957) reviewed all the studies in English and German up to that time. Unfortunately, no real quantitative data are provided, follow-up periods varied from childhood through to adulthood, and there were already signs of slippage away from schizophrenia to autism and any type of severe disorder. The best that can be said of this review is that the majority of cases of true EOS were considered to have a poor prognosis, and onset in childhood particularly so. The review by Werry (1979), which added two more studies, reached similar conclusions. The best of these two studies was the one by Bennett and Klein (1966) in which subjects were first seen 30 years previously and diagnosed using adult-type schizophrenic symptoms. All but one of 14 were still in hospital (or had died there) and were grossly disabled. The clinical state was by then indistinguishable from adults similarly institutionalized.

There are four more or less acceptable studies (in English) of long-term outcome of EOS since 1970—from Sweden (Gillberg et al. 1993), Germany (Eggers 1978, 1989; Schmidt 1995), and New Zealand (Werry et al. 1991). Two U.S. studies (Jordan and Prugh

1971; King and Pittman 1971) and one from the United Kingdom (Howells and Guirguis 1984) had to be rejected because of the impossibility of disentangling schizophrenia from autism, organic disorders, and bipolar disorder at index or outcome. The total number of subjects is just over 200, although not all were seen at follow-up. The study by Eggers (1978) is the only one in which the majority of subjects had childhood onset and is vague in many details. Also, 11 years later (Eggers 1989), over a quarter of subjects were rediagnosed as having schizoaffective disorder, although this did not influence outcome greatly. One study (Werry et al. 1991) has a substantial minority of child-onset cases, but the other two (Gillberg et al. 1993; Schmidt 1995) are exclusively adolescent-onset or nearly so. Intervals of follow-up vary from 1 to many years, but the majority of subjects were seen at late adolescence or beyond.

The implications of this study are fairly clear: most subjects have one or more further psychotic episodes, acute hospitalization is frequent during these, and a variable majority (over two-thirds) remain sufficiently handicapped as to be unemployable and dependent on parents or the state. Most of these subjects are seriously impaired. The studies use global judgments about outcome status (fair, good, etc.) so that variations in proportions are likely subjective in nature. Diagnosis of schizophrenia at outcome is somewhat more variable— ranging from at least one-third (Gillberg et al. 1993) through the majority (Eggers 1978, 1989; Schmidt 1995; Werry et al. 1991). A variable minority are rediagnosed, mostly as having bipolar or schizoaffective disorder (Eggers 1989; Werry et al. 1991). A few have no psychiatric diagnosis, but even these may be quite disabled (e.g., Gillberg et al. 1993), and this suggests that they may actually have had schizophrenic residual states.

It is commonly held that the outcome in EOS is worse than in adult-onset schizophrenia, although, as Gillberg et al. (1993) point out, this may be to some degree an artifact of longer duration of illness. Werry et al. (1991) felt that outcome in EOS was only marginally worse than in adults; but M. H. Schmidt (personal communication, 1995) found significantly greater disability (in negative symptoms) than in a comparable adult group. Thus, outcome in childhood-onset schizophrenia probably is somewhat worse—but to an unknown degree

Treatment and Other Factors in Outcome

Treatment

There are no studies of the effect of treatment on long-term outcome in EOS. There is some preliminary evidence (see Campbell et al. 1993; McClellan and Werry 1992) that antipsychotic drugs may have somewhat similar beneficial short-term effects in children and adolescents as they do in adults, but data are too few to make firm conclusions.

Other Factors

Again, there has been little study of this treatment, and the results are not always consistent. Eggers (1978) found onset before age 10 and poor premorbid personality, and Werry et al. (1991) found poor premorbid adjustment, older age at onset, delusions, flat affect, degree of impairment after first admission, and length of follow-up as predictive of a poorer outcome. M. H. Schmidt (personal communication, 1995) found only degree of recovery from the first episode and number of subsequent episodes as predictive. Gillberg et al. (1993) did not analyze predictors of outcome separately for mood and schizophrenic psychoses. In summary, as in adults, premorbid personality and degree of recovery from the first episode/admission are probably predictive, but the other prognostic indicators in adults—gender (Iacono and Beiser 1992) and age at onset (DeLisi 1992)—are unclear. This may be due to early onset being indicative of an etiologically more homogeneous "congenital" group (DeLisi 1992; Murray et al. 1992).

Current Work on Treatment and Outcome

It is only in the last few years that research on schizophrenia in children and adolescents seems to have attracted renewed interest (see Asarnow and Asarnow 1994). The National Institute of Mental Health is actively encouraging such research, which currently covers outcome, pharmacotherapy, neurobiology, and symptomatology, but there are still no more than a handful of researchers.

Summary

Schizophrenia in children and adolescents is qualitatively similar to that in adults. However, most of those afflicted will become severely disabled adults, and it is probable that outcome is somewhat worse than in adults. Variables (except premorbid personality) influencing outcome are unclear. Despite the fact that schizophrenia is to a significant degree—especially in males—a disorder of adolescence, research into EOS per se is very limited. This clearly needs correction.

▼ Bipolar Mood Disorder

Bipolar illness requires that the patient have at least one manic episode—that is, a distinct period of abnormality characterized by elevated, expansive, or irritable mood with distinctive symptoms of grandiosity, decreased sleep, pressured speech, flight of ideas, distractibility, increased activity, and/or hedonistic behavior. Some patients have only manic attacks, some have both manic and depressive attacks, and some have mixed features during any one episode.

There is reason to believe that bipolar disorder has been underdiagnosed in children and adolescents and that it has been misdiagnosed as schizophrenia (Carlson 1990; Weller et al. 1986; Werry et al. 1991) or sometimes as hyperactivity (Carlson 1990; Varanka et al. 1988). One reason for confusion with schizophrenia is that onset in adolescence is more likely to be flagrantly psychotic than in adults (McGlashan 1988).

There are very few follow-up studies of early-onset bipolar disorder into adulthood, but those that exist are uniform in showing that the disorder resembles that in adults—that is, there is a strong tendency for further episodes—although the risk reported varies from 90% to 40% (Gillberg et al. 1993; Strober et al. 1995; Werry et al. 1991). The more favorable figures may reflect better compliance with lithium prophylaxis (see Strober et al. 1990) in specialist centers or shorter follow-up periods, because the risk of recurrence increases with time until it finally stabilizes (Goodwin and Jamison

1990). As in adults, the overall level of adjustment is better than in schizophrenia (Werry et al. 1991), although this was not so in one study (Gillberg et al. 1993). Despite this, the level of disability (continued dependency) seems to be quite high in at least 50% of cases (Gillberg et al. 1993; Werry et al. 1991). However, comparative data suggest that contrary to expectation, early-onset cases do no worse than those of adult onset (Carlson 1990; McGlashan 1988).

One study of 23 mostly adolescent-onset cases (Werry and McClellan 1992) showed that intelligence and premorbid function were the best predictors with gender (males worse) and positive family history (worse) weakly so. Strober et al. (1995) found that, as in adults, patients with mixed and cycling forms had more relapses. Predictive studies are complicated by the fact that they can study the effect only of variables that have been measured at index, and these tend to vary from study to study.

In summary, studies of bipolar disorder in children and adolescents are few in number and complicated by the risk of misdiagnosis as schizophrenia. Results suggest that many will go on to have the disorder as adults. The exact number who will do so and the predictors of outcome remain to be elucidated. The prognosis does not appear to be very different from that in adults.

▼ Odd or Eccentric Children

Recent reviews (Gillberg 1991; Meijer and Treffers 1991; Petti and Vela 1990; Wolff 1991a, 1991b) document the long-standing interest in the field of child psychiatry in a group of children whose social-interactional development, cognitive development, and/or neurodevelopment are grossly disordered but who are not autistic, schizophrenic, or merely mentally retarded nor merit other diagnoses (except comorbidly). Unfortunately, the reviews also demonstrate the nosological chaos in their studies, with such children having been variously described as being atypical, borderline (see Logfren et al. 1991; Petti and Vela 1990), or schizophrenic (Bender 1947; Cantor 1982); as having schizophrenia spectrum disorder (Asarnow et al. 1991); as being "schizoid" (Wolff 1991a); and, most recently, as having Asperger's "autistic psychopathy" (see Gillberg 1991; Wolff 1991a, 1991b) or multiple complex developmental disorder (Towbin et al. 1993). There also seems no doubt that some of these groups are contaminated with truly psychotic children (see Petti and Vela 1990). There has been argument as to whether these children are part of the autistic or the schizophrenic spectrum of disorders or whether their disorders are related to borderline personality disorder (see Gillberg 1991; Logfren et al. 1991; Meijer and Treffers 1991; Petti and Vela 1990; Szatmari et al. 1989).

There has also been a continued suspicion that there is some relationship in some cases with brain damage/dysfunction (Cantor 1982; Fish et al. 1992; Nagy and Szatmari 1989). Some may have a kind of juvenile organic personality syndrome, although others have the type of neurodevelopmental delays and aberrations (e.g., Gordon et al. in press; Towbin et al. 1993) that are now recognized as risk factors for schizophrenia and schizotypal disorder (see Asarnow et al. 1991; Murray et al. 1992; Walker et al. 1991). The high-risk-for-schizophrenia studies (Erlenmeyer-Kimling et al. 1993; Fish et al. 1992) have shown that schizophrenia in a parent greatly increases the risk of producing such a child.

Fortunately, but coincidentally, DSM-III began the process of trying to separate clearly for adults three of the main streams in this group, into borderline (BPD), schizotypal (STPD), and schizoid personality disorders. The creation of strictly defined Asperger's syndrome may also help. However, these subdivisions are too recent (and may not be entirely valid) to be as helpful as they may ultimately become. Nevertheless, there are some intimations of what long-term outcome may be and what kind of research is needed to clarify this.

Such children have an increased risk of becoming schizophrenic but seldom do so (Gillberg 1991; Logfren et al. 1991; Petti and Vela 1990; Wolff 1991a; Wolff et al. 1991). The risk for this is highest in children with a schizophrenic relative (Erlenmeyer-Kimling et al. 1993; Fish et al. 1992) or who are odd, present late in childhood, and are definitely not autistic (Wolff 1991b).

There is a high frequency of continued impaired adjustment in adult life, although studies are too vague and too few to state exactly how many or what the best predictors are. The degree of this

impairment varies greatly and is most centered on intimate relationships and dependency (Logfren et al. 1991), but is not necessarily
incompatible with a career or marriage (Wolff 1991b).

What psychiatric diagnoses these children or adolescents will
have as adults is unclear, although there are four possibilities. The
first possibility is STPD. This is best established and predicted by
having a parent with schizophrenia (Erlenmeyer-Kimling et al. 1993;
Fish et al. 1992; Wolff 1991a) and a cluster of childhood symptoms
of unusual fantasies and special interests (imaginative preoccupations); being described as a loner and showing developmental delays
or aberrations (such as learning disorders, dyspraxias, etc.); and presenting in middle childhood rather than earlier (Wolff 1991b). In
short, the children in this group have probably met most of the
diagnostic criteria for STPD but have not hitherto been diagnosed
as such (Tantam 1988b, 1988c) because there are very few studies
of STPD in children (Nagy and Szatmari 1989). This is confirmed
by Wolff's (1991b) careful retrospective rediagnosis from the original case records of her 32 subjects.

The second possible psychiatric diagnosis such children or adolescents will have as adults is schizoid personality disorder. Used
strictly, as in DSM, these individuals lack the schizophreniform
"positive" symptomatology (such as unusual fantasies and hypersensitivity) and are characterized mostly by a lack of interest in interpersonal relationships. It has been posited (Rutter 1989; Szatmari
1992) that this could be one of the late outcomes of autistic spectrum disorders. Wolff et al. (1991) were unable to confirm this, but
their sample was mostly STPD (Tantam 1988b, 1988c) and contained only three autistic spectrum cases. Tantam (1988b, 1988c)
looked at 60 adults with lifelong eccentricity and social isolation
and found that those with autistic spectrum disorders (including
Asperger's) differed from those with schizoid disorder in having
neurodevelopmental histories and symptoms. Thus, this outcome
remains plausible but requires further study.

BPD is the third possible psychiatric diagnosis. Unfortunately,
the widespread former use of the term *borderline child* is most confusing because such children are severely handicapped in social interaction and have much more in common with children who are
schizoid or who have schizotypal disorder (see Logfren et al. 1991).

Although it is commonly assumed that properly diagnosed border-line personality–type children and adolescents will breed true in adulthood, there is as yet no evidence by which to assess this (Meijer and Treffers 1991; Petti and Vela 1990). In addition to the above three possibilities, other diagnoses should not be excluded as possibilities at this stage.

In summary, there is evidence to suggest that seriously odd, eccentric children do not often grow out of their problems but that they are a diagnostically heterogeneous group, and that diagnoses in the spectra of autistic, Asperger's, schizoid, schizotypal, and border-line disorders have different outcomes. Better outcome studies using strict diagnostic criteria derived from modern nosology (DSM-IV and ICD-10) are sorely needed.

▼ Summary

This review has been concerned with a group of disorders that are characterized by gross defects in a child's abilities for reality testing (psychoses) and/or to form intimate relationships. These defects are such that these children or adolescents are set conspicuously apart from their peers. They comprise a variety of disorders, some of which, by definition, always have a childhood onset and others of which are well-recognized in adults, from whom the diagnostic criteria and labels accrue. Research into long-term outcome varies in quantity and quality but it seems that, although most affected individuals show some degree of improvement, these disorders do not go away, but continue to have devastating and lasting effects on social and often on cognitive development as well. The result for many is a lifelong handicap, especially in the capacity to form intimate relationships or to become independent. Generally speaking, too, adult-type disorders seen in childhood breed true into adulthood.

Developments in both nosology and research methods now allow these disorders to be subject to the kind of investigation that their degree of chronic handicap merits. Clearly, too, the idea that some of these disorders are adult disorders is incorrect, and the focus in many should now shift to their origins in childhood and adolescence.

The need to focus on development of more effective and comprehensive treatment approaches, which may include pharmacotherapeutic and intellectual, behavioral, social, and familial psychotherapeutic interventions, is clearly there. The cross-fertilization between child and adult psychiatry would be useful in developing more effective treatment strategies and would help in delineating factors that influence long-term outcome. Child and adolescent psychiatrists may need to redirect their priorities in research away from areas that are important (such as sexual abuse, child advocacy, custody disputes, parenting, psychotherapy, and family therapy) but that, unlike the severely handicapping disorders reviewed here, are not biological in etiology or in potential remedy and hence can be pursued as well by nonmedical investigators.

▼ References

American Psychiatric Association: Diagnostic and Statistical Manual of Mental Disorders, 2nd Edition. Washington, DC, American Psychiatric Association, 1968

American Psychiatric Association: Diagnostic and Statistic Manual of Mental Disorders, 3rd Edition. Washington, DC, American Psychiatric Association, 1980

American Psychiatric Association: Diagnostic and Statistic Manual of Mental Disorders, 3rd Edition, Revised. Washington, DC, American Psychiatric Association, 1987

American Psychiatric Association: Diagnostic and Statistic Manual of Mental Disorders, 4th Edition. Washington, DC, American Psychiatric Association, 1994

Andreasen NC, Carpenter WT: Diagnosis and classification of schizophrenia. Schizophr Bull 19:199–214, 1993

Andreasen NC, Flaum M: Schizophrenia: the characteristic symptoms. Schizophr Bull 17:27–50, 1991

Asarnow RF, Asarnow JR (eds): Childhood onset schizophrenia. Schizophr Bull 20:591–746, 1994

Asarnow JR, Asarnow RF, Hornstein N, et al: Childhood-onset schizophrenia: developmental perspectives on schizophrenic disorders, in Schizophrenia: A Life-Course Developmental Perspective. Edited by Walker EF. New York, Academic Press, 1991, pp 97–123

Beitchman JH: Childhood schizophrenia: a review and a comparison with adult-onset schizophrenia. Psychiatr Clin North Am 8:793–814, 1985

Bender L: Childhood schizophrenia: clinical study of 100 schizophrenic children. Am J Orthopsychiatry 17:40–45, 1947

Bennett S, Klein H: Childhood schizophrenia: thirty years later. Am J Psychiatry 122:1121–1124, 1966

Campbell M, Green WH: Pervasive developmental disorders of childhood, in Comprehensive Textbook of Psychiatry, 4th Edition. Edited by Kaplan HI, Sadock BJ. Baltimore, MD, Williams & Wilkins, 1985, pp 1680–1683

Campbell M, Gonzalez NM, Ernst M, et al: Antipsychotics (neuroleptics), in Practitioner's Guide to Psychoactive Drugs for Children and Adolescents. Edited by Werry JS, Aman MG. New York, Plenum, 1993, pp 269–296

Cantor S: The Schizophrenic Child: A Primer for Parents and Professionals. Montreal, Canada, Eden Press, 1982

Carlson GA: Child and adolescent mania: diagnostic considerations. J Child Psychol Psychiatry 31:331–342, 1990

DeLisi LE: The significance of age of onset for schizophrenia. Schizophr Bull 18:209–216, 1992

DeMyer MK, Hingtgen JN, Jackson RK: Infantile autism reviewed: a decade of research. Schizophr Bull 7:388–451, 1981

Eggers C: Course and prognosis in childhood schizophrenia. J Autism Dev Disord 8:21–36, 1978

Eggers C: Schizoaffective psychoses in childhood: course and prognosis in childhood schizophrenia. J Autism Dev Disord 19:327–342, 1989

Eisenberg L: The course of childhood schizophrenia. Archives of Neurology and Psychiatry 78:69–83, 1957

Erlenmeyer-Kimling L, Cornblatt BA, Rock D: The New York High Risk Project: anhedonia, attentional deviance and psychopathology. Schizophr Bull 19:141–153, 1993

Fish B, Marcus J, Hans SL, et al: Infants at risk for schizophrenia: sequelae of a genetic neurointegrative defect. Arch Gen Psychiatry 49:221–235, 1992

Freeman BJ, Ritvo ER, Needleman R, et al: The stability of cognitive and linguistic parameters in autism: a five-year prospective study. J Am Acad Child Adolesc Psychiatry 24:459–464, 1985

Gillberg C: Diagnosis and Treatment of Autism. New York, Plenum, 1989

Gillberg IC: Outcome in autism and autistic-like conditions. J Am Acad Child Adolesc Psychiatry 30:375–382, 1991

Gillberg IC, Steffenburg S: Outcome and prognostic factors in infantile autism and similar conditions: a population-based study of 46 cases followed through puberty. J Autism Dev Disord 17:273–287, 1987

Gillberg IC, Wahlstrom J, Forsman A, et al: Teenage psychoses: epidemiology, classification and reduced optimality in the pre-, peri- and neonatal periods. J Child Psychol Psychiatry 27:87–98, 1986

Gillberg IC, Hellgren L, Gillberg C: Psychotic disorders diagnosed in adolescence: outcome at age 30 years. J Child Psychol Psychiatry 34:1173–1186, 1993

Goodwin FK, Jamison KR: Manic-Depressive Illness. New York, Oxford University Press, 1990

Gordon CT, McKenna K, Giedd J, et al: Childhood-onset schizophrenia: neurobiological characterization and pharmacologic response: NIMH studies in progress. Schizophr Bull 20:697–712, 1995

Howells JG, Guirguis WR: Childhood schizophrenia 20 years later. Arch Gen Psychiatry 41:123–128, 1984

Iacono WG, Beiser M: Where are all the women in first-episode studies of schizophrenia? Schizophr Bull 18:471–480, 1992

Jordan K, Prugh DC: Schizophreniform psychoses of childhood. Am J Psychiatry 128:323–331, 1971

Kafantaris V, Ernst M, Samuel R, et al: Psychotic disorders in hospitalized adolescents: diagnostic issues. Paper presented at the 39th annual meeting of the American Academy of Child and Adolescent Psychiatry, Washington, DC, October 1993

Kanner L: Autistic disturbances of affective contact. Nervous Child 2:217–230, 1943

Kanner L: Childhood psychoses: a historical overview. Journal of Autism and Childhood Schizophrenia 1:14–19, 1971a

Kanner L: Followup study of 11 autistic children originally reported in 1943. Journal of Autism and Childhood Schizophrenia 1:119–145, 1971b

King LJ, Pittman GD: A follow-up of 65 adolescent schizophrenia patients. Diseases of the Nervous System 32:328–334, 1971

Knobloch H, Pasamanick B: Some etiological and prognostic factors in early infantile autism and psychosis. Pediatrics 55:182–191, 1975

Kobayashi R, Murata T, Yoshinga K: A follow-up study of 201 children with autism in Kyushi and Yamaguchi areas in Japan. J Autism Dev Disord 22:395–412, 1992

Kolvin I: Studies in the childhood psychoses, I: diagnostic criteria and classification. Br J Psychiatry 118:381–384, 1971

Logfren DP, Bemporad J, King J, et al: A prospective follow-up study of so-called borderline children. Am J Psychiatry 148:1541–1547, 1991

Lotter V: Factors related to outcome in autistic children. Journal of Autism and Childhood Schizophrenia 4:263–277, 1974

Malhotra S, Singh SP: Disintegrative psychosis of childhood: an appraisal and case study. Acta Paedopsychiatr 56:37–40, 1993

McClellan JM, Werry JS: Schizophrenia in pediatric psychopharmacology. Psychiatr Clin North Am 15:131–148, 1992

McClellan JM, Werry JS, Ham M: A follow-up study of early onset psychosis: comparison between outcome diagnosis of schizophrenia, mood disorders and personality disorders. J Autism Dev Disord 23:243–262, 1993

McGlashan TH: Adolescent versus adult onset of mania. Am J Psychiatry 145:221–223, 1988

Meijer M, Treffers PDA: Borderline and schizotypal disorders in children and adolescents. Br J Psychiatry 158:205–212, 1991

Mesibov GB: Current perspectives and issues in autism and adolescence, in Autism in Adolescents and Adults. Edited by Schopler E, Mesibov GB. New York, Plenum, 1983, pp 37–53

Murray RM, O'Callaghan E, Castle DJ, et al: A neurodevelopmental approach to the classification of schizophrenia. Schizophr Bull 18:319–332, 1992

Nagy J, Szatmari P: A chart review of schizotypal personality disorders in children. J Autism Dev Disord 16:351–367, 1989

Petti TA, Vela RM: Borderline disorders of childhood: an overview. J Am Acad Child Adolesc Psychiatry 29:327–337, 1990

Prior M, Werry JS: Autism, schizophrenia and allied disorders, in Psychopathological Disorders of Childhood, 3rd Edition. Edited by Quay HC, Werry JS. New York, Wiley, 1986, pp 156–210

Rumsey JM, Rappoport JL, Sceery WR: Autistic children as adults: psychiatric, social and behavioral outcomes. J Am Acad Child Adolesc Psychiatry 24:465–473, 1985

Rutter M: Childhood schizophrenia reconsidered. Journal of Autism and Childhood Schizophrenia 2:315–337, 1972

Rutter M: Infantile autism and other pervasive developmental disorders, in Child and Adolescent Psychiatry: Modern Approaches, 2nd Edition. Edited by Rutter M, Hersov L. Oxford, England, Blackwell, 1985a, pp 545–566

Rutter M: The treatment of autistic children. J Child Psychol Psychiatry 26:193–214, 1985b

Rutter M: Child psychiatric disorders in ICD-10. J Child Psychol Psychiatry 30:499–514, 1989

Rutter M, Schopler E: Classification of pervasive developmental disorders: some concepts and practical considerations. J Autism Dev Disord 22:459–482, 1992

Strober M, Morrell W, Lampert C, et al: Relapse following discontinuation of lithium maintenance therapy in adolescents with bipolar I illness: a naturalistic study. Am J Psychiatry 147:457–461, 1990

Strober M, Schmidt-Lackner S, Freeman R, et al: Recovery and relapse in adolescents with bipolar affective illness: results from a five-year naturalistic, prospective followup. J Am Acad Child Adolesc Psychiatry 34:724–731, 1995

Szatmari P: The validity of autistic spectrum disorders: a literature review. J Autism Dev Disord 22:583–600, 1992

Szatmari P, Bartolucci G, Brenner R, et al: A follow-up study of high-functioning autistic children. J Autism Dev Disord 19:213–225, 1989

Tantam D: Asperger's syndrome. J Child Psychol Psychiatry 29:245–256, 1988a

Tantam D: Lifelong eccentricity and social isolation, I: psychiatric, social and forensic aspects. Br J Psychiatry 153:777–782, 1988b

Tantam D: Lifelong eccentricity and social isolation, II: Asperger's syndrome or schizoid personality disorder? Br J Psychiatry 153:783–791, 1988c

Towbin KE, Dykens EM, Pearson GS, et al: Conceptualizing "borderline syndrome of childhood" and "childhood schizophrenia" as a developmental disorder. J Am Acad Child Adolesc Psychiatry 32:775–782, 1993

Tsai LY: Is Rett syndrome a subtype of pervasive developmental disorders? J Autism Dev Disord 22:551–562, 1992

Varanka TM, Weller RA, Weller EB, et al: Lithium treatment of manic episodes with psychotic features in prepubertal children. Am J Psychiatry 145:1557–1559, 1988

Volkmar FR: Childhood disintegrative disorder: issues for DSM-IV. J Autism Dev Disord 22:625–642, 1992

Volkmar FR, Cohen DJ: Comorbid association of autism and schizophrenia. Am J Psychiatry 12:1705–1708, 1991

Walker EF, Davis DM, Gottlieb LA, et al: Developmental trajectories in schizophrenia: elucidating the divergent pathways, in Schizophrenia: A Life-Course Developmental Perspective. Edited by Walker EF. New York, Academic Press, 1991, pp 299–331

Weller RA, Weller EB, Tucker SG, et al: Mania in prepubertal children: has it been underdiagnosed? J Affect Disord 11:151–154, 1986

Werry JS: The childhood psychoses, in Psychopathological Disorders of Childhood, 2nd Edition. Edited by Quay HC, Werry JS. New York, Wiley, 1979, pp 43–89

Werry JS: Child and adolescent (early onset) schizophrenia: a review in the light of DSM-III-R. J Autism Dev Disord 22:601–624, 1992

Werry JS, McClellan JM: Predicting outcome in child and adolescent (early onset) schizophrenia and bipolar disorder. J Am Acad Child Adolesc Psychiatry 31:147–150, 1992

Werry JS, McClellan JM, Chard L: Child and adolescent schizophrenia, bipolar and schizoaffective disorder: a clinical and outcome study. J Am Acad Child Adolesc Psychiatry 30:457–465, 1991

Wing L: Autistic adults, in Diagnosis and Treatment of Autism. Edited by Gillberg C. New York, Plenum, 1989, pp 419–432

Wing L, Gould J: Severe impairments of social interaction and associated abnormalities in children: epidemiology and classification. J Autism Dev Disord 9:11–29, 1979

Wolff S: Schizoid personality in childhood and adult life, I: the vagaries of diagnostic labelling. Br J Psychiatry 159:615–620, 1991a

Wolff S: Schizoid personality in childhood and adult life, III: childhood picture. Br J Psychiatry 159:629–635, 1991b

Wolff S, Townshend R, McGuire RJ, et al: Adult adjustment and the continuity with schizotypal personality disorder. Br J Psychiatry 159:620–629, 1991

World Health Organization: The International Classification of Diseases (ICD-8), 8th Revision. Geneva, Switzerland, World Health Organization, 1968

World Health Organization: The ICD-10 Classification of Mental and Behavioural Disorders: Clinical Descriptions and Diagnostic Guidelines. Geneva, Switzerland, World Health Organization, 1992

Chapter 10

Childhood Speech and Language Disorders

Joseph H. Beitchman, M.D., F.R.C.P.C., D.A.B.P.N., and E. B. Brownlie, B.Sc.

Empirical research provides compelling evidence for an association between speech and language impairment and psychiatric disorder in childhood. This association is not surprising given the centrality of language to human communication and development. To provide a diagnostically comprehensive assessment and a therapeutically effective approach to treatment, clinicians working with children require an understanding of the intimate relationship between speech and language impairment and psychiatric disorder.

This chapter provides an overview of the long-term outcome of speech and language disorders in childhood. It will be of interest to

The assistance of Beth Wilson, B.Sc., in the preparation of this manuscript is gratefully acknowledged.

students, researchers, and clinicians. The chapter begins with a definition of terms and a review of peak ages at onset of speech and
language disorders followed by a discussion of the epidemiological
literature. A summary of the psychiatric disorders associated with
speech and language impairment and the long-term outcome of
childhood speech and language impairment concludes the chapter.

▼ Definitions

Language is a systematic means of communication. As social beings,
language is integral to human life—our thoughts, feelings, actions,
and accumulation of knowledge. The grammar of language is a set
of rules that defines the system of signals used to communicate
ideas. Grammar includes phonology, syntax, semantics, and pragmatics. Phonology describes how to combine sounds into words;
syntax describes how to combine words into sentences; semantics
describes the meaning of words and sentences; and pragmatics
describes how to participate in a conversation, how to sequence
sentences, and how to anticipate information required by a listener.
Language is used to signal needs, intentions, and feelings. It is also
used for self-talk and the mediation of thought processes. In broad
terms, language is differentiated into expressive and receptive
forms. Expressive language includes speech, or the articulation of
sounds. Receptive language refers to the understanding of what has
been heard.

▼ Speech and Language Disorders

Childhood speech disorders include problems in speech production, which may reflect stuttering or voice abnormalities. Speech
production difficulties are due to an inability to articulate sound
segments even if there is no disorder in the ability to follow the
rules of the sound system, either in production or discrimination.
Such disorders may occur in healthy children, or in those children
with other developmental disabilities such as autism, mental retardation, or hearing impairment.

Childhood language disorders may involve impairment in the central cognitive processes associated with syntax, semantics, or pragmatics. These processes are component parts of linguistic functioning, and include auditory memory, comprehension, discrimination, and integration.

Language impairment is a heterogeneous condition. For example, language impairment may involve problems with auditory comprehension, phonological discrimination, syntax, or all three. Unless the precise nature of the deficit can be specified, it is impossible to know which linguistic function or group of functions may be affected.

A number of researchers have attempted to define distinct linguistic impairments among children identified as having speech and language disorders. Fundudis et al. (1979) identified three different groups of language-delayed children. However, these identifications were based on the age at which the child achieved different motor milestones, and the presence or absence of medical conditions, such as cerebral palsy, autism, and others. Other researchers have defined distinct linguistic subtypes among those with speech and language impairments. Wolfus et al. (1980), using a very small clinic sample, identified two groups of language-impaired children: one group was impaired in the production of syntax and phonology, and the other group was impaired in phonological discrimination, digit span, and semantics. Cantwell et al. (1980) described a group of children with pure speech problems and another group with language-processing problems. Beitchman et al. (1989) described four groups of children obtained from a community sample: children showing poor auditory comprehension but performing normally on other language tests, children displaying poor articulation but performing normally on other language tests, children with impaired performance on a variety of expressive and receptive language tests, and children performing above average on a variety of language tests.

Age at Onset

Typically, speech and language disorders are among the earliest signs of developmental dysfunction. The first peak in the detection of speech and language disorders occurs in infancy. Delayed onset of speech sounds may be the most obvious symptom. The child may show little evidence of babbling, cooing, and other forms of proto-language indicative of speech and language development. The child may show various speech sound substitutions or articulation errors. Many speech sound substitutions are developmentally appropriate. For instance, the 3-year-old who says "wabbit," instead of "rabbit," is employing speech sound substitutions that are developmentally appropriate. Identifying children whose speech or language functioning is developmentally inappropriate or whose speech or language functioning does not develop within a normal range of time may require an assessment by a speech and language pathologist. In addition, the child may demonstrate grammatical immaturities, for instance by using a statement form with a rising intonation to indicate a question rather than using the more mature interrogative. A child who asks, "Have cookie, please?" where "please" ends in a rising intonation, compared with "Can I have a cookie, please?" shows immaturities in grammar.

Problems of comprehension are more subtle and can begin in infancy. Although the child may not speak or may have very limited expressive language, one expects comprehension to exceed spoken language. Diagnosing language comprehension disorders or delays is difficult. Comprehension delays should be suspected in any child with autisticlike symptoms, or any child who seems "spacey," lost, or odd.

A second peak in the detection of speech and language problems occurs during the preschool years. Often, preschool teachers and other caregivers may detect speech and language problems that parents fail to notice. By comparison with the speech and language functioning of the child's peer group, speech and language problems may be more easily detectable. Since behavioral problems and symptoms associated with attention deficit disorder frequently co-occur with speech and language impairment, these problems are often first identified during the preschool years. Often the third year of life is used as a measuring stick for children's speech and language functioning. Commonly, parents do not seek speech and language assessments for their children before that age. This waiting period also contributes to the preschool years as a peak period for detection of speech and language problems.

The third peak occurs on formal entry to kindergarten. The more formalized nature of a school setting increases expectations of the child's language abilities. The child must now be able to attend to story time, follow more complex oral instructions, and verbally express his or her own wants and needs. Under these demanding circumstances, problems with auditory memory and auditory discrimination may manifest for the first time. The child may have difficulty communicating effectively and, consequently, may shy away from interactions requiring verbal expression. In addition, the child may become restless and fidgety, leading teachers to identify him or her as having a behavior problem.

▼ Epidemiology

Numerous authors have estimated a broad range of speech and language disorder prevalence rates from 3% to 15% (Fundudis et al. 1979; Jenkins et al. 1980; Silva et al. 1983; Stanovich 1982). Generally, these prevalence rates are based on surveys of preschool-aged children due to the typical age at onset of speech and language problems. Stevenson and Richman (1976) estimated a 3.1% prevalence rate for expressive language delay among 705 3-year-old children. Fundudis et al. (1979), surveying the health records of 3,300 children, calculated a 4% rate of language delay.

Jenkins et al. (1980) used a community sample to determine the types of behavior problems found in preschool-aged children. They found that 36 out of 168 children (21.6%) between the ages of 2 and 5 years displayed probable or definite speech *and* language problems as defined by standardized language tests.

Silva et al. (1983) surveyed language problems in a community sample of 3-year-old children. They defined language delay as deficits in verbal comprehension, expression, or both, as measured by a standardized language test. Using this definition, they reported a 7.6% prevalence rate for language delay in their sample of 1,027 children.

Beitchman et al. (1986b) reported higher prevalence rates in their community survey of 5-year-old children. Using standardized speech and language tests, they reported a prevalence rate of 19% for speech and/or language disorders.

Discrepancies among prevalence rates are a function of sample selection (such as varying age ranges as opposed to community versus clinic samples), measurement techniques, and the types of disorders being investigated as well as how they are operationalized (Beitchman 1985). A review of language intervention literature found that over a 6-year period a great deal of variability between articles on standardization and comprehensiveness of language assessment procedures existed (Werner and Smith 1982). This variability is reflected in the types of speech and language disorders assessed and reported and the prevalence figures cited. Beitchman et al. (1986b) found that when cut-off scores for defining disorder were adjusted to reflect one or two standard deviations (SD) from the mean, prevalence rates of speech and language disorders in 5-year-old children dropped from 19% (one SD below the mean) to 9.6% (two SD below the mean).

▼ Speech and Language Impairment and Psychiatric Disorders

Sufficient data demonstrate that children with speech and language impairments are at increased risk for developing psychiatric disorders of all kinds (Baker and Cantwell 1987; Beitchman et al. 1986a; Cantwell and Baker 1977, 1985, 1991; Chess and Rosenburg 1974; Grinnell et al. 1983; Gualtieri et al. 1983; Kotsopoulis and Boodoosingh 1987; Stevenson and Richman 1976). Whether one samples from a psychiatric population or a language-impaired population, it is clear that language impairment and psychiatric disorders occur together.

Although there are fairly extensive data with regard to the prevalence of speech and language impairment and its association with psychiatric disorders, the specific types of linguistic impairment associated with various psychiatric disorders have not yet been catalogued. In the following section, specific psychiatric disorders and the corresponding linguistic deficit(s) are described. For some conditions, specific relationships are identified; for others, only general statements are possible.

Hyperactivity

There is good evidence that attention-deficit hyperactivity disorder (ADHD) is associated with language impairment. Beitchman et al. (1986a) reported a prevalence of 30% ADHD in their sample of 5-year-old children with language impairments. Baker and Cantwell (1987) found hyperactivity to be the preponderant diagnosis among children with language impairments. Using empirical clustering techniques, Beitchman et al. (1989) were able to show not only that ADHD was the most common psychiatric diagnosis, but that ADHD was associated with global deficits in speech and language functioning. Speech and language deficits included articulation, language comprehension, and language expression.

Emotional Disorders

Socioemotional disorders are also more prevalent among language-impaired children than among children in control groups. Beitchman et al. (1986a) reported a 12.8% prevalence rate of emotional disorders among language-impaired children compared with 1.5% among children in control groups. The differences in prevalence rates were particularly marked among females when teacher reports of emotionality were considered. Baker and Cantwell (1987) found an association between language impairment, emotional disorder, and being female. Tallal et al. (1989) found that preschool girls with language impairments scored significantly higher on the social withdrawal scale of the Child Behavior Checklist (Achenbach and Edelbrock 1983) than did girls in control groups. For reasons as yet unknown, girls with language impairments seem to be more prone to emotional disorders than boys with language impairments.

Elective Mutism

Some recent evidence suggests that children with elective muteness may be delayed in the onset of language and may show immaturities in communication (especially articulation) as late as 6–10 years of age (Kolvin and Fundudis 1981; Lerea and Ward 1965).

Children who overcome their elective mutism may continue to show speech and language impairment.

In a review of 24 cases of elective mutism, Kolvin and Fundudis (1981) found delayed speech milestones, articulation disorders, electroencephalographic immaturities, and associated developmental problems of soiling and enuresis. Mild cognitive delays have also been found in children initially diagnosed as electively mute (Parker et al. 1960; Reed 1963). Wilkin (1985), in a study comparing 24 subjects who had elective muteness with control subjects, found that one-third of the subjects with elective muteness had delayed speech development or problems with articulation. Although speech and language immaturities may not be a necessary precondition for elective mutism, they coexist in about one-third to one-half of cases (Kolvin and Fundudis 1981; Wilkin 1985). These immaturities appear to be a logical precursor to elective mutism and may play some causal or contributory role.

Learning Disabilities

Learning disabilities are a heterogeneous group of disorders in which children's educational performance falls below that expected on the basis of IQ, and the performance deficits cannot be attributed to inadequate instruction. Often, learning disabilities are also referred to as dyslexia. Three models of dyslexia have been described: an auditory verbal subtype, a visuospatial subtype, and a mixed subtype. The auditory verbal subtype is considered the most prevalent.

Commonly, children with speech and language impairment have academic problems; the reported prevalence rates range from 45% (Baker and Cantwell 1987) to 90% (Stark et al. 1984). Conversely, children with learning disabilities often exhibit speech and language problems (Benton 1975; Vellutino 1979). Barkley (1981) reported that 60% of children with reading disabilities had associated language disorders. Deficits in specific aspects of linguistic functioning among children with reading disabilities, including verbal encoding and labeling, are common (Denckla and Rudel 1976; Vellutino et al. 1975).

Recently, phonological processing (the use of phonological information in the processing of written and oral language) has been reported as an important causal factor in the acquisition of reading skills (Wagner and Torgesen 1987). It is also known that phonological processing is highly correlated with general measures of language function, such as educational attainment and visuospatial abilities (Lewis et al. 1989). Consequently, one would expect to find increased rates of reading disabilities and educational failure among individuals with speech and language impairments.

Several investigators have noted that the more pervasive the speech and language impairment, the worse the academic outcome in terms of reading ability tends to be (Childs and Angst 1984; Silva et al. 1987). Furthermore, in a group of 3- to 11-year-old children with reading disabilities, language skills were reported to decline with age. The authors viewed this decline as a partial result of the children's reading difficulties (Share and Silva 1987).

Autism

Disturbances of language and communication have long been held to be one of the hallmarks of autism. Most children with autism show delays in the development of language, with comprehension deficits being especially marked (Lord 1984; Tager-Flusberg 1981). Abnormalities in the use of language are associated with autism throughout childhood, and autistic children are usually unable to use language in a flexible and reciprocal conversational manner.

It is important to recognize that some of the language behaviors associated with autism, such as echolalia and delayed echolalia, are understandable within the context of developmental communicative behavior. Prizant and Wetherby (1986) described a developmental sequence of intentional communicative behavior, suggesting that immediate and delayed echolalia can be understood as transitional phenomena toward communicative language. Controlling for receptive language age, the language and communication of autistic children may not be demonstrably different from those of developmental-receptive dysphasic individuals, for instance. A study comparing sentence comprehension strategies of autistic, language-impaired, and unimpaired subjects found that children with autism and those with language impairment responded to a sentence comprehension task in a manner similar to that used by unimpaired children at similar levels of comprehension ability. It appears that the language-processing deficits seen in autism may be less unique to the syndrome than previously believed (Paul et al. 1988). The differences in language and communication between developmental-receptive dysphasic individuals and autistic individuals may be a matter of degree, and as Prizant and Wetherby (1986) suggest, a possible manifestation of the developmental level of intentional communicative social behavior.

Differences in mental age (Siegel et al. 1989) or receptive language age (Sigman and Ungerer 1984) can account for differences between autistic individuals and mentally retarded individuals. The studies of Bartak et al. (1975) and Bartak and Rutter (1974) are commonly cited as showing differences in the language and communication of autistic and dysphasic individuals; however, these studies compared groups that were not equivalent in receptive language age. Despite the vast literature on language disturbances in autism, the specific and unique features of these disturbances remain to be defined.

▼ Outcome

The association between speech and language development on the one hand and concurrent academic achievement and psychiatric disorders on the other has been described in the first part of this chapter. However, the long-term outcome of speech and language impairment is not well known, nor are the long-term academic and psychiatric consequences of early speech and language impairment. To fully appreciate the implications of speech and language impairment, it will be necessary to understand their outcome in the related domains of academic achievement and psychiatric disorders.

This section is organized in three parts: speech and language outcomes, psychiatric and behavioral disorders, and learning disabilities. Many of the same studies report on one or more of these outcome dimensions, but for the sake of clarity, studies will be referred to more than once to include the specific outcomes of interest described in each of the identified three sections.

Speech and Language Outcome

The follow-up of preschool children with language impairments has recently been reviewed by Aram and Hall (1989). These authors identified 20 studies that examined aspects of the long-term outcome of speech and language disorders. Of the 20 studies reviewed, only two (Hall and Tomblin 1978; King et al. 1982) described outcome to adulthood. The remaining were outcome studies to early and middle childhood, and in one study (Aram et al. 1984), to early adolescence.

The two studies of adult outcome, reporting that communication problems continued in 50%–67% of cases at follow-up, are retrospective reports (Hall and Tomblin 1978; King et al. 1982). There were no independent assessments of speech and language development at follow-up (only the vague term *communication problems*), and no information was provided about the specifics of the original speech and language delays. The samples were nonrepresentative; in one study only 36 of the original cohort of 281 children were found at follow-up (Hall and Tomblin 1978), and in the second study only 50 of the original 150 children were found at follow-up (King et al. 1982). A third study of the adolescent outcome of speech and language impairments reported by Aram et al. (1984) did provide more details of the children's speech and language development both initially and at follow-up. However, the entire sample consisted of 20 subjects, of whom 25% were found to be retarded, thus limiting the generalizability of the findings.

Other studies of the outcome of language-impaired children have been noted, but the findings are consistent with those reported by Aram and Hall (1989). For example, Sheridan and Peckham (1975) report that 71% of 11-year-old children who had marked speech defect at 7 years were in need of special education or had speech problems.

Bishop and Edmundson (1987a) reported that 63% of their sample of 87 4-year-olds continued to show language deficits when assessed at 5.5 years of age. The poor outcome group at 5 years showed significantly lower language scores than the good outcome group when followed to 8.5 years. Baker and Cantwell (1987) reported on the 5-year outcome of children attending a speech and hearing clinic. These authors found that 85% of the children continued to show some form of speech or language problem at follow-up.

Generalizations drawn from the literature are limited by the heterogeneous nature of the groups studied and the frequent failure to report important subject parameters, as well as the widespread variability in outcome measures reported (Aram and Hall 1989). The clinic-based studies reported continued speech and/or language problems in 40%–88% of their cases. However, clinic cases are subject to referral biases, limiting generalizability of findings. Furthermore, few studies tested the children at follow-up and instead depended on secondary sources, such as parents, for evidence of communication problems. In addition, retrospective studies were based on incomplete testing of the children at the time of the original assessment. The true rate of recovery of speech and language impairment can only be obtained from community studies utilizing representative random selection methods with well-defined criteria and appropriate controls.

Silva et al. (1987) conducted an important community study of 3-year-old children with speech and language disorders. Although they followed these children to age 11 and beyond, and reported on IQ, reading achievement, and behavior problems at follow-up, they did not provide systematic information on the outcome of the children's speech and language development after age 7. At the age of 7, however, 2% were found to have general delays in language, 2.8% specific expressive delays, and 3.6% specific comprehension delays for a total of 8.4% for any language delay. Forty percent with delays at age 3 were delayed at age 5, and 31.4% delayed at age 5 were delayed at age 7. General language delays continued in 52%–79% of those with general language delays 2–4 years later.

Using a randomly selected community sample of 5-year-old children, Beitchman et al. (1994) conducted a 7-year follow-up study of the stability and outcome of speech and language development. Speech and language problems appeared fairly stable over time. Seventy-two percent of children who were impaired at age 5 were still impaired at 12.5 years. Sixty-five percent of cases with speech-only problems and 72% of cases with language-only problems continued to show speech and language impairment at follow-up. Eighty-one percent of the children with both speech *and* language problems at 5 years continued to manifest speech and language impairment at 12.5 years.

Children with both speech and language problems had the poorest outcomes in the sample: 81% continued to exhibit a speech and/or language problem at follow-up. Similarly, children with both receptive and expressive impairment were more likely to continue to be language impaired than were children with a history of only expressive or receptive impairment or children with normal language (Beitchman et al. 1994). These findings are consistent with the idea that children with more pervasive problems show poorer outcomes compared with children with isolated problems (Bishop and Edmundson 1987a).

What can one conclude from this? Because the findings reported by Beitchman et al. (1994) are based on a careful epidemiological sample of 5-year-old children who had not yet been identified as language impaired, it is likely that the base rate (19%–35%) of recovery to preadolescence can be predicated upon these rates. In any speech and language clinic, more severely impaired youngsters of various ages are likely to be seen, and consequently the recovery rates would be expected to be lower. Additionally, there is evidence that in some language-impaired samples, nonverbal IQ is an important predictor of eventual language performance (Aram et al. 1984; Griffiths 1969). Disorders confined to speech or the phonological aspects of language have a more favorable outcome than disorders involving other or more general aspects of language (Beitchman et al. 1994; Hall and Tomblin 1978; King et al. 1982).

Finally, in very young children (2- to 3-years-old), transient language deficits may be distinguished from persistent language deficits by the following characteristics: the smaller the child's vocabulary, the more irregular the child's eating, and the less time engaged in quiet activities with mother, the more persistent the expected language deficit will be (Fischel et al. 1989). The age at which the initial assessment is made and the age at which follow-up occurs will also determine the rate of recovery of speech and language problems. The proportion of language-impaired children with good out-comes will be much lower in samples using older children than in those using younger children.

Psychiatric and Behavioral Disorders

Although there are reports describing the outcome and natural history of childhood speech and language impairment, much less is known about the longitudinal course of the associated psychiatric disorder so often concurrently present. This is surprising given that childhood speech and language disorders are highly prevalent (Baker and Cantwell 1987; Beitchman et al. 1986b), that speech and language disorders are associated with high rates of psychiatric morbidity (Baker and Cantwell 1987; Beitchman et al. 1986a; Cohen et al. 1993), and that much has been published on the topic of speech and language impairment.

Follow-up studies of psychiatric disorders among children with severe language impairments are uncommon. Only two follow-up studies have been located in which the psychiatric status of severely language-impaired children has been examined.

In a follow-up study (the number of years was unspecified by the authors) of 14 children with a history of atypical developmental aphasia with autistic features (ADLD) and 14 children at least 2.5 years of age with developmental language disorder (DLD) who were not speaking or were speaking very poorly, Paul et al. (1983) revealed that only 12% developed near-normal language. The DLD group with good comprehension showed the most consistent progress. In both the ADLD group and the DLD group, children whose comprehension exceeded expression often made gains in sociability and showed the most consistent progress in expressive language.

In a report on the 2- to 3-year outcome of 14 boys with developmental receptive aphasia initially assessed at an average age of 95 months, Cantwell et al. (1989) found that half of the dysphasic children were communicating well, but some of the dysphasic children had developed increased difficulties in peer relationships. These authors raised questions regarding the traditional view that the socioemotional problems are simply secondary features that develop in response to the social difficulties associated with language disability. Contrary to what they seemed to believe at the outset of their study, they wondered if the social deficits constitute a basic part of developmental receptive language disorder.

These two studies described the language and psychiatric outcomes of language-impaired children with known psychiatric disorders. What about the psychiatric outcome of speech- and language-impaired children unselected for psychiatric or behavioral problems?

In a follow-up study of 8-year-old children originally seen at age 3, Stevenson et al. (1985) found that "low language structure" at age 3 predicted behavioral deviance at 8. When behavioral deviance at age 3 was controlled, low language structure still predicted behavioral deviance. The definition of low language structure included approximately 25% of the 3-year-olds and was not considered to reflect extreme problems.

Comprehensive language and psychiatric assessments were conducted in a follow-up study by Baker and Cantwell (1987). The overall prevalence of psychiatric disorders in their clinic sample of speech- and language-impaired children increased from 44% initially to 60% at 5-year follow-up. They noted a trend toward an association between lack of improvement in speech and language functioning and the development of a psychiatric disorder. Although one cannot generalize from this study to the population at large because the sample was originally selected from a speech and hearing clinic, nevertheless it does indicate the high psychiatric morbidity rate among speech- and language-impaired children followed over 5 years.

The Dunedin community study (Silva et al. 1987) showed the long-term association of language delays at 3 years with behavioral deviance at age 11. The groups with general language delay and with comprehension delay had significantly higher scores on behavior problem scales than the group with expressive language delays. Further, when IQ, reading scores, family disadvantage, and sex were controlled statistically, the association with behavior problems was reduced but remained significant. What is not known from this study is whether these findings would be significant with less severe language delays. Recall that Silva et al. (1987) defined language delays as scores at or below the fifth percentile and selected subjects representing the bottom 2%–3% of their sample.

Benasich et al. (1993) also controlled socioeconomic status (SES) and performance IQ and found language impairment at age 4 to be associated with behavior problems at age 8; among girls, expressive language at age 4 significantly predicted social withdrawal scores on the Child Behavior Checklist at age 8. Interestingly, neither concurrent language functioning nor the severity of speech and language disorder at age 4 was related to behavioral problems at age 8, again with SES and IQ controlled.

Similarly, Beitchman et al. (in press) reported that speech and language status at 5 years was a better predictor of psychiatric outcome at 12.5 years than was concurrent speech and language functioning. Early speech impairment and early language impairment were associated with higher rates of psychiatric disorder at follow-up, compared with children with no speech or language impairment. Furthermore, rates of disorder were not significantly higher for children who remained speech and language impaired compared with children whose speech and language status improved at follow-up. These findings highlight the impact of speech and language problems, even when they appear to improve over time. Why should early speech and language problems be associated with later psychiatric disorder even when such problems improve? The secondary effects of early speech and language problems may be so enduring that they continue despite the subsequent improvement in speech and language competence. School failure and poor peer relations could be examples of problems that, once established, set in motion a sequence of events that lead to, or increase the risk for, the development of psychiatric disorder. It is also possible that the association between psychiatric disorder and early speech and language impairment is related to associated social disadvantage or adversity rather than being related to the speech and language impairment itself. Under these circumstances, the associated disadvantage could continue to age 12.5 even when the speech and language impairment does not. Alternatively, it may be that the effects of an earlier disadvantage are so enduring (e.g., deprivation during a sensitive period) that they carry forward in time even if the disadvantage is mitigated and the speech and/or language functioning improves.

These findings seem to suggest that remediation of speech and language impairment in preschoolers is not sufficient to protect against the later development of psychiatric disorder. Whatever causative factors are set in motion along with or due to the speech and language impairment, their effects will need to be redressed if the risk of psychiatric disorder is to be reduced.

Speech and language disorders may result in specific types of psychiatric problems that change over time. Five-year-old children with speech and language impairments were more likely to be diagnosed with ADHD and emotional disorders than were children in control groups, but there was no difference in the rate of conduct disorders between these two groups (Beitchman et al. 1986a). At follow-up, significant differences no longer appeared in the rates of ADHD, but emotional disorders were significantly more common among the speech- and language-impaired group than among the control group (Beitchman et al., in press).

J. H. Beitchman and colleagues (unpublished observations) found that at 12.5 years, mothers rated boys with a prior history of speech and language impairment as being significantly more immature, hostile, and withdrawn than boys in control groups. Teachers rated these boys as unpopular and immature. Girls with a prior history of language impairment were described by their teachers as more socially withdrawn and depressed and by their mothers as more immature/hyperactive and depressed/withdrawn than girls in control groups.

In a 28-year follow-up of 24 subjects initially scoring more than 1.5 SD below the mean on the Peabody Individual Achievement Test (PIAT), a prekindergarten test of articulation, Felsenfeld et al. (1992) revealed that they scored significantly worse than control subjects on articulation, expressive language, and receptive language. On a questionnaire measure of personality, both groups scored well within the normal range for the dimensions of extroversion and introversion.

Although of interest, the report by Felsenfeld et al. (1992) has major limitations. First, no information is provided on the language competence of the subjects originally tested in prekindergarten. The measure used at the inception of that study only tested articulation; consequently, the level of language competence of these children is unknown. Secondly, the Eysenck Personality Inventory was administered when the subjects were in the 11th grade (approximately 17–18 years old), although other tests of language and cognition were given to the subjects as adults. Consequently, it is not known how valid these personality measures are for teenagers nor is it known to what extent the findings at 17–18 can be extrapolated to 32- to 34-year-olds.

The middle childhood and young adolescent outcome of early language impairment shows clearly the increased risk of psychiatric and behavioral problems. The risk was increased when receptive language was more severely compromised than expressive language. For children with language comprehension problems, the psychiatric outcomes seemed to affect social relations more so than other behavioral dimensions. Children with more pervasive problems were at higher risk for psychiatric problems than those with more circumscribed problems. For instance, the risk of psychiatric disorder associated with speech delays was lower than that associated with language delays. Psychiatric disorder was associated with early speech and language delays even when such delays improved. Although there is evidence that a history of speech and language delays in early childhood increases the risk of psychiatric disorder in middle and later childhood, there is virtually no information on the outcome to adulthood.

Learning Disabilities

Given that learning disabilities (LD) are known to be associated with speech and language impairment, it is of interest to determine to what extent speech and language impairment in early childhood constitutes a risk for the later development of LD.

Because few studies actually define LD, reports that mention the number of children requiring special education, who are achieving below grade level or who have some kind of learning disorder have been included.

In a follow-up study of 190 of 215 11-year-old children who had appreciable "unintelligibility of speech" at 7 years, Sheridan and Peckham (1975) report that 71% were judged to be in need of special education treatment or to have speech problems. Aram and Nation (1980) reexamined 63 children who had been identified as language impaired before the age of 5. At the age of 9, 40% presented learning problems. Many were in special classes for learning-disabled or mentally retarded children.

Aram et al. (1984) found that of 20 adolescents originally assessed 10 years earlier as preschoolers with language delays, 20% had IQ scores on the Wechsler Intelligence Scale for Children—Revised (WISC-R) in the mentally deficient range, and 69% of the remaining 16 children required special education tutoring, grade retention, or LD class placement. Stark et al. (1984) found that 90% of language-impaired children showed some form of reading disability at follow-up 3–4 years later at the age of 12.

Baker and Cantwell (1987) found that one-quarter of their sample of 300 children from a speech and hearing clinic developed a learning disorder during the interval to follow-up. A history of speech or language disorders was found to increase the risk for learning disorders, which appeared after an initial period of apparently normal school achievement. The children most at risk for the development of learning disorders were those children with some impairments in language. Seventy-one percent of children who developed a learning disorder had a language disorder initially, compared with only 54% of those without a learning disorder. The children with language comprehension disorders were most likely to develop a learning disorder.

Silva et al. (1987) identified three types of language delay in 3-year-olds: expressive language delay, delayed comprehension, and general language delay. Analyses at age 11 revealed that all three groups increased their reading scores at a significantly slower rate than the remainder of the sample without language delay.

The study by Beitchman et al. (1993) was the only follow-up community study to use well-defined groups of language-impaired and learning-disabled children. LDs were defined with and without a correction for the child's IQ (Beitchman et al. 1993).

Among 12.5-year-old children with a history of preschool speech and language impairment, compared with a matched control group, the increased odds of having an LD at age 12.5, using the battery composite from the Kaufman Test of Educational Achievement

(Kaufman and Kaufman 1985), ranged from 3.3, when an achievement IQ discrepancy score was used to define LD, to 14, when achievement below grade level irrespective of IQ was used to define LD.

By use of the IQ corrected definition of LD, the best preschool predictors of LD were Wechsler Preschool and Primary Scale of Intelligence (WPPSI) full-scale IQ, scores on the Bankson screening test of expressive language, the screening test for the auditory comprehension of language, and visual motor skills. One of the strongest predictors ($P< 0.0001$) of LD was a less than eighth grade maternal education.

Children identified at age 5 with a speech and language disorder are at significantly increased risk for LDs compared with children without language impairment. Not all the increased risk of LDs is necessarily due to the speech and language impairment. Some of this increased risk is attributable to factors such as lower IQ, lower SES, lower maternal education, and birth status (second or later born), which are associated with speech and language impairment. However, speech and language impairment remained an independent predictor of LD, even after controlling for these other variables (Beitchman et al. 1993).

▼ Summary

Speech and language disorders are common and are associated with considerable morbidity. This includes increased rates of ADHD, as well as LDs and emotional disorders, such as anxiety and depression. The reason for the increased rates of psychiatric disorders among the children with speech and language impairments has generated many hypotheses. It is possible that children with speech and language impairments have some increased vulnerability based on a maturational lag (Bishop and Edmundson 1987b) or neurodevelopmental deficits (Beitchman 1985; Beitchman et al. 1989; Tallal et al. 1989). In the presence of additional risks such as certain temperamental characteristics or an inhospitable or insensitive environment, psychiatric disorders develop. It is also possible that the speech and language impairment acts secondarily through such phenomena as school failure, peer rejection, and scapegoating, which in turn lead to behavioral disturbance. There may also be cognitive impairments based on the speech and language disturbance that limit the child's ability to use language to modulate emotions, express feelings and ideas, delay action, and control his or her own and other people's behavior. Under these circumstances, the child will be prone to behavioral outbursts on the one hand and withdrawal on the other. The complex mechanisms that mediate the relation between speech and language impairment and psychiatric problems are poorly understood and clearly in need of further investigation.

The etiology of speech and language impairment is unknown but associated with such variables as large family size, lower SES, later-born status, and hearing impairment. In addition, there is suggestive evidence that familial and genetic factors are implicated in the transmission of speech and language impairment. Birth and pregnancy variables, medical disorders suggestive of organic brain damage, and mental retardation are also known to be associated with speech and language impairment (Beitchman et al., in press).

Although there have been many reports (of variable quality) on the short-term and intermediate outcome of speech and language delays, there are no methodologically acceptable studies on the adult outcome of speech and language impairment. Clearly, those studies reporting on outcomes to middle childhood and early adolescence demonstrate substantial levels of morbidity in speech and language development, behavioral adjustment, and learning. To what extent these difficulties continue into adulthood and affect vocational outcome, psychosocial functioning, and mental health more generally is not yet known but should be the subject of future enquiry.

The evidence to date does not permit firm conclusions on the association between speech and language impairment and specific psychiatric disorders. There is evidence showing the association of speech and language impairment with ADHD (Baker and Cantwell 1992; Beitchman et al. 1989). However, it is not known if this association is specific to a younger population or if it also applies to adolescents and to adults. It is not known if this association is related to aspects of intelligence such as low verbal IQ or some other cognitive function such as auditory processing (Cook et al. 1993). The report by Benasich et al. (1993) with 8-year-old children did not

confirm the association of language impairment and ADHD. Beitchman et al. (in press) failed to show an increased incidence of ADHD
at age 12.5 among their sample of children who were speech and
language impaired at age 5. However, they did find a significantly
increased rate of ADHD at age 12.5 among concurrently language-
impaired boys compared with boys with normal speech and language
functioning at follow-up.

Evidence implicates low verbal IQ as a predictor of conduct
disorder and delinquent behavior. These findings have repeatedly
been the subject of research reports (e.g., Hinshaw 1992; Lynam et
al. 1993; Moffitt 1990). The basis for the association between low
verbal IQ and conduct disorder is not known, but the possibility
that executive functions are compromised in these youngsters has
been suggested (Moffitt 1990). It is also not known to what extent
preschool speech and language impairment is a precursor of low
verbal IQ, conduct disorder, and juvenile delinquency. Because executive function deficits have also been implicated in ADHD
(Barkley 1990; Schachar and Logan 1990), and because ADHD is
known to be a correlate of conduct disorder and delinquency, it is
possible that the increased risk for ADHD and conduct disorder
among language-impaired children is due to a common underlying
impairment in executive functions. At this time these ideas seem
most fruitfully thought of as promising hypotheses worthy of further
investigation.

The practitioner needs to be alert to speech and language problems for many reasons. Many children thought to be willfully disobedient, oppositional, or hyperactive may have problems with
auditory memory, auditory discrimination, or auditory comprehension. Unless these deficits are recognized, attempts to treat these
children may be misplaced and may end in failure. The language
skills of withdrawn, depressed children also need to be examined
because language deficits are found among children with emotional
disorders. These deficits may intensify poor peer relations and tendencies to social isolation. The clinician should always suspect language comprehension problems in any child who seems odd, who
says things that appear out of context, or who seems spacey or autisticlike. The proper planning of the child's academic program de-
pends on an appropriate understanding of the child's linguistic

capabilities. Psychotherapeutic encounters must of necessity be in tune with the child's language skills in order to be maximally beneficial and effective. It is possible that many psychotherapeutic failures can be traced to unrecognized language impairments.

Given the persistent nature of speech and language impairment and the high rates of associated psychiatric morbidity, continued research into the etiology, treatment, and prevention of speech and language impairment and associated disorders is strongly encouraged. Although early intervention programs utilizing enriched language environments now exist for young children at high risk, the effects of these types of programs remain insufficiently studied and inadequately understood. It is difficult to confidently describe the specific outcomes of speech and language intervention (Nye et al. 1987) or the effects of language intervention on coexisting behavior problems. Careful evaluation and long-term follow-up are essential to properly assess the effects of these types of programs. This information is of practical and theoretical importance; it will assist in directing scarce treatment resources and will aid in clarifying the relation between language impairment and psychiatric disorders.

▼ References

Achenbach TM, Edelbrock CS: Manual for the Child Behavior Checklist and Revised Child Behavior Profile. Burlington, VT, University of Vermont, 1983

Aram DM, Hall NE: Longitudinal follow up of children with preschool communication disorders: treatment implications. School Psychology Review 18:487–501, 1989

Aram DM, Nation JE: Preschool language disorders and subsequent language and academic difficulties. Journal of Communication Disorders 13:159–170, 1980

Aram DM, Ekelman BL, Nation JE: Preschoolers with language disorders: 10 years later. Journal of Speech and Hearing Research 27:232–244, 1984

Baker L, Cantwell DP: A prospective psychiatric follow up of children with speech/language disorders. J Am Acad Child Adolesc Psychiatry 26:546–553, 1987

Barkley R: Learning disabilities, in Behavioral Assessment of Childhood Disorders. Edited by Mash E, Terdal L. New York, Guilford, 1981, pp 441–482

Barkley R: Attention Deficit Hyperactivity Disorder: A Handbook for Diagnosis and Treatment. New York, Guilford, 1990

Bartak L, Rutter M: Use of personal pronouns by autistic children. Journal of Autism and Childhood Schizophrenia 4:217–222, 1974

Bartak L, Rutter M, Cox A: Comparative study of infantile autism and specific developmental receptive language disorder, I: the children. Br J Psychiatry 126:127–145, 1975

Beitchman JH: Speech and language impairment and psychiatric risk: toward a model of neurodevelopmental immaturity. Psychiatr Clin North Am 8:721–735, 1985

Beitchman JH, Nair R, Clegg M, et al: Prevalence of psychiatric disorders in children with speech and language disorders. J Am Acad Child Psychiatry 25:528–535, 1986a

Beitchman JH, Nair R, Clegg M, et al: Prevalence of speech and language disorders in 5 year old kindergarten children in the Ottawa Carleton region. Journal of Speech and Hearing Disorders 51:98–110, 1986b

Beitchman JH, Hood J, Rochon J, et al: Empirical classification of speech/language impairment in children, II: behavioral characteristics. J Am Acad Child Adolesc Psychiatry 28:118–123, 1989

Beitchman JH, Ferguson B, Schachter D, et al: A seven year follow up of speech/language impaired and control children: final report. Toronto, Canada, Health and Welfare Canada, 1993

Beitchman JH, Brownlie EB, Inglis A, et al: Seven year follow up of speech/language impaired and control children: speech/language stability and outcome. J Am Acad Child Adolesc Psychiatry 33:1322–1330, 1994

Beitchman JH, Wild J, Kroll R: An overview of childhood speech and language disorders, in Basic Handbook of Child Psychiatry. Edited by Noshpitz J. New York, Wiley (in press)

Beitchman JH, Brownlie EB, Inglis A, et al: Seven year follow up of speech/language impaired and control children: psychiatric outcome. Journal of Child Psychology (in press)

Benasich AA, Curtiss S, Tallal P: Language, learning, and behavioral disturbances in childhood: a longitudinal perspective. J Am Acad Child Adolesc Psychiatry 32:585–593, 1993

Benton AL: Developmental dyslexia: neurological aspects, in Advances in Neurology. Edited by Friedlander WJ. New York, Raven, 1975, pp 1–47

Bishop DVM, Edmundson A: Language impaired 4 year olds: distinguishing transient from persistent impairment. Journal of Speech and Hearing Research 52:156–173, 1987a

Bishop DVM, Edmundson A: Specific language impairment as a maturational lag: evidence from longitudinal data on language and motor development. Dev Med Child Neurol 29:442–459, 1987b

Cantwell DP, Baker L: Psychiatric disorder in children with speech and language retardation: a critical review. Arch Gen Psychiatry 34:583–591, 1977

Cantwell DP, Baker L: Psychiatric and learning disorders in children with communication disorders, II: methodological approach and findings, in Advances in Learning and Behavioral Disabilities, Vol 4. Edited by Gadow KD. Greenwich, CT, JAI, 1985, pp 29–47

Cantwell DP, Baker L: Association between attention deficit hyperactivity disorder and learning disorders. Journal of Learning Disabilities 24:88–95, 1991

Cantwell D, Baker L, Mattison R: Psychiatric disorders in children with speech and language retardation: factors associated with development. Arch Gen Psychiatry 37:423–426, 1980

Cantwell D, Baker L, Rutter M, et al: Infantile autism and developmental receptive dysphasia: a comparative follow up into middle childhood. J Autism Dev Disord 19:19–31, 1989

Chess S, Rosenburg M: Clinical differentiation among children with initial language complaints. Journal of Autism and Childhood Schizophrenia 4:99–109, 1974

Childs PJ, Angst DM: Description of an ongoing special education preschool program. Language, Speech and Hearing Services in Schools 15:262–266, 1984

Cohen NJ, Davine M, Horodezky N: Unsuspected language impairment in psychiatrically disturbed children: prevalence and language and behavioral characteristics. J Am Acad Child Adolesc Psychiatry 32:595–603, 1993

Cook JR, Mausbach T, Burd L, et al: A preliminary study of the relationship between central auditory processing disorder and attention deficit disorder. J Psychiatry Neurosci 18:130–137, 1993

Denckla MB, Rudel R: Naming of pictured objects by dyslexic and other learning disabled children. Brain Lang 39:1–15, 1976

Felsenfeld S, Broen PA, McGue M: A 28 year follow up of adults with a history of moderate phonological disorder: linguistic and personality results. Journal of Speech and Hearing Research 35: 1114–1125, 1992

Fischel J, Whitehurst G, Caulfield M, et al: Language growth in children with expressive language delay. Pediatrics 82:218–227, 1989

Fundudis T, Kolvin I, Garside R: Speech Retarded and Deaf Children: Their Psychological Development. New York, Academic Press, 1979

Griffiths C: A follow up study of children with disorders of speech. British Journal of Disorders of Communication 4:46–56, 1969

Grinnell SW, Scott-Hartnet D, Glasier JL: Language disorders. J Am Acad Child Adolesc Psychiatry 22:580–581, 1983

Gualtieri CT, Koriath W, Van Bourgondien M, et al: Language disorders in children referred for psychiatric services. J Am Acad Child Adolesc Psychiatry 22:580–581, 1983

Hall PK, Tomblin JB: A follow up study of children with articulation and language disorders. Journal of Speech and Hearing Disorders 63:220–226, 1978

Hinshaw SP: Externalizing behavior problems and academic underachievement in childhood and adolescence: causal relationships and underlying mechanisms. Psychol Bull 111:127–155, 1992

Jenkins S, Bax M, Hart H: Behavior problems in preschool children. J Child Psychol Psychiatry 21:5–17, 1980

Kaufman AS, Kaufman NL: Kaufman Test of Educational Achievement. Circle Pines, MN, American Guidance Service, 1985

King RR, Jones C, Laskey E: In retrospect: a fifteen year follow up report of speech and language disordered children. Language, Speech, and Hearing Services in Schools 13:24–32, 1982

Kolvin I, Fundudis T: Elective mute children: psychological development and background factors. J Child Psychol Psychiatry 22:219–232, 1981

Kotsopoulos A, Boodoosingh L: Language and speech disorders in children attending a day psychiatric programme. British Journal of Disorders of Communication 22:227–236, 1987

Lerea L, Ward D: Speech avoidance among children with oral communication defects. J Psychol 60:265–270, 1965

Lewis BA, Ekelman BL, Aram DM: A familial study of severe phonological disorders. Journal of Speech and Hearing Research 32:713–724, 1989

Lord C: Language comprehension and cognitive disorder in autism, in Cognitive Development in Atypical Children. Edited by Siegel L, Morrison FJ. New York, Springer-Verlag New York, 1984, pp 67–82

Lynam D, Moffitt T, Stouthamer-Loeber M: Explaining the relation between IQ and delinquency: class, race, test motivation, school failure, or self control? J Abnorm Psychol 102:187–196, 1993

Moffitt TE: The neuropsychology of conduct disorder. Development and Psychopathology 5:135–151, 1993

Nye C, Foster SH, Seaman D: Effectiveness of language intervention with the language/learning disabled. Journal of Speech and Hearing Disorders 52:348–357, 1987

Parker EB, Olsen TF, Throckmorton MC: Social casework with elementary school children who do not talk in school. Social Work 5:64–70, 1960

Paul R, Cohen DJ, Caparulo BK: A longitudinal study of patients with severe developmental disorders of language learning. J Am Acad Child Psychiatry 22:525–534, 1983

Paul R, Fischer ML, Cohen DJ: Brief report: sentence comprehension strategies in children with autism and specific language disorders. J Autism Dev Disord 18:669–679, 1988

Prizant BM, Wetherby AM: Communicative intent: a framework for understanding sociocommunicative behavior in autism. J Am Acad Child Adolesc Psychiatry 26:472–479, 1986

Reed GF: Elective mutism in children: a reappraisal. J Child Psychol Psychiatry 4:99–107, 1963

Schachar R, Logan G: Impulsivity and inhibitory control in normal development and childhood psychopathology. Developmental Psychology 26:710–720, 1990

Share DL, Silva PA: Language deficits and specific reading retardation: cause or effect? British Journal of Disorders of Communication 22:219–226, 1987

Sheridan MD, Peckham C: Follow up at 11 years of children who had marked speech defects at 7 years. Child: Care, Health and Development I:157–166, 1975

Siegel B, Vukicevie J, Elliot CR, et al: The use of signal detection theory to assess DSM-III-R criteria for autistic disorder. J Am Acad Child Adolesc Psychiatry 28:542–548, 1989

Sigman M, Ungerer JA: Cognitive and language skills in autistic, mentally retarded, and normal children. Developmental Psychology 20:293–302, 1984

Silva PA, McGee RO, Williams SM: Developmental language delay from three to seven years and its significance for low intelligence and reading difficulties at age seven. Dev Med Child Neurol 25:783–793, 1983

Silva PA, Williams SM, McGee RO: A longitudinal study of children with developmental language delay at age three: later intelligence, reading and behaviour problems. Dev Med Child Neurol 29:630–640, 1987

Stanovich K: Individual differences in the cognitive processes of reading, I: word decoding. Journal of Learning Disabilities 15:485–493, 1982

Stark RE, Bernstein LE, Condino R: Four year follow up study of language impaired children. Annals of Dyslexia 34:50–69, 1984

Stevenson J, Richman N: The prevalence of language delay in a population of three year old children and its association with general retardation. Dev Med Child Neurol 18:431–441, 1976

Stevenson J, Richman N, Graham P: Behaviour problems and language abilities at three years and behavioural deviance at eight years. J Child Psychol Psychiatry 26:215–230, 1985

Tager-Flusberg H: On the nature of linguistic functioning in early infantile autism. J Autism Dev Disord 11:45–46, 1981

Tallal P, Dukette D, Curtiss S: Behavioral/emotional profiles of preschool language impaired children. Development and Psychopathology 1:51–67, 1989

Vellutino FR: Dyslexia: Theory and Research. Cambridge, MA, MIT Press, 1979

Vellutino RR, Smith H, Steger JA, et al: Reading disability: age differences and the perceptual deficit hypothesis. Child Dev 46: 487–493, 1975

Wagner RK, Torgesen JK: The nature of phonological processing and its causal role in the acquisition of reading skills. Psychol Bull 101:192–212, 1987

Werner EE, Smith RS: Vulnerable but not Invincible: A Longitudinal Study of Resilient Children and Youth. New York, McGraw Hill, 1982

Wilkin R: A comparison of elective mutism and emotional disorders in children. Br J Psychiatry 146:198–203, 1985

Wolfus B, Moscovitch M, Kinsbourne M: Subgroups of developmental language impairment. Brain Lang 10:152–171, 1980

Chapter 11

Clinical Issues in Longitudinal Research

Gabrielle Weiss, M.D., F.R.C.P.C.

W riting this chapter is a privilege because it will enable me to systematize the vast amount of information gained in carrying out a 15-year prospective follow-up study on 100 hyperactive children. This study was carried out together with colleagues, initially John S. Werry and Klaus Minde and for the last 10 years of the study with Lily Hechtman; the results of this longitudinal research were summarized and published in a book, *Hyperactive Children Grown Up* (Weiss and Hechtman 1993). Sharing the lives of 70–100 hyperactive children along with 46 matched healthy control subjects during their childhood, adolescence, and adulthood taught us many things over and above the research information we sought, which was the course and outcome of attention-deficit hyperactivity disorder (ADHD) in children. Some of these ways of understanding our probands and how they coped, often creatively, with difficulties at different ages came to us incidentally from our long-term contact with them in the course of the study. For myself, it was through carrying out this longitudinal research that I feel I learned the major part of my child and adult psychiatry. I learned about the developmental processes of healthy and troubled children and the ingenuity of many individuals at all ages in finding adaptive mechanisms, whereas others floundered because of their circumstances. What at one time were pathological symptoms sometimes became special abilities in some children or adults; a case illustration of this is described for clarification.

In clinical practice we may come to know a child or an adult more or less intensely over a given period of time. After the treatment is ended we often lose touch with them, particularly if they are doing well. By contrast, in prospective follow-up studies, in which we follow and systematically assess subjects at predetermined regular intervals (whether the individuals are currently troubled or not), we obtain a different perspective on the different pathways of growth and development over a much longer period of time. We can observe how the symptoms of a given syndrome affect the developmental process at different ages, and how incidental life changes such as divorce of parents, other crises, school situations, and the appearance for the individual of a new significant person in their life can significantly worsen or improve the course of the disorder.

Because the professional engaged in a prospective longitudinal study often sees the same individual over many years, he or she becomes a part of the life of that person (child or adult) even without offering any treatment to them. As a "participant observer," the researcher may positively affect the individual. In our prospective follow-up study we capitalized on this by having the same psychiatrist follow the individual involved at every assessment. The advantages and disadvantages of this from a clinical and research standpoint will be discussed.

▼ Development of Intimacy

Those of us who were involved in the prospective longitudinal study, which continued over 15 years with annual and later assessments every 5 years lasting 2–3 days, have experienced the power of this intimacy. It meant that we could travel 3,000 miles and interview a subject in jail, and the person readily confided his or her life story, including crimes for which the subject was never caught. It also meant meeting a subject in another city in a hotel room, spending the day together in this unlikely setting, with the subject entrusting his or her life story to us without reservation and usually looking forward to the contact with positive anticipation.

The clinical value of this long-term close relationship was the mutual satisfaction and the trust that developed, which allowed the sharing of a wealth of confidential information not obtained on structured rating scales administered to the same individual by a research assistant unknown to the subject. The disadvantage from a research standpoint is the impact of this relationship on the subject. As previously mentioned, the researcher becomes a participant observer who by his or her presence over time may positively influence the person being studied. The advantages seemed to us to outweigh the disadvantages, in that a more realistic appraisal of the subjects' self-esteem and real functioning could be obtained. Self-rating scales were sometimes not valid, especially when insight was lacking.

▼ The Issue of Healthy Control Subjects

It is essential that a longitudinal study employ either a matched healthy control group or a matched patient comparison group; without such a group any findings of outcome are not valid. Following the healthy control subjects as closely as the probands using the same methodology was what first taught us about the myth of normality. Our control group should have been "supernormal." We selected children matched on age, IQ, socioeconomic class, and gender who had had no troubles according to their teachers and parents in their academic work and behavior at school or at home. They were otherwise selected randomly by choosing a child in the same classroom as the proband whose name was closest in the alphabet to the first letter in the last name of the proband. As we followed these supposedly "supernormal" children we soon discovered that they too had difficulties. In adulthood one or two developed major depression and schizophrenia. It was because of the pathology also present in the healthy control subjects that ADHD was not a predictor of adult bipolar disorders or schizophrenia. We recognized *normality* to be a relative term, with almost nobody going through development without some problems.

▼ The Use of Confidential Information

Although we sought to keep information confidential, from the research point of view, we had no predetermined idea of what to do with some of the confidential information about which we learned. We traced one subject whom we discovered was being sought across Canada by the police for a serious crime. We learned incidentally about the suicidal risk of some subjects whom did not wish treatment. In the end, we made every attempt to "save life" and used every means at our disposal to do this. When we received reports of repeated drunken driving we tried and usually succeeded in getting help for the person involved.

The ambiguous aspect of our role was highlighted when a subject clearly required treatment but was unwilling to see anyone but ourselves. We would offer crisis intervention and use this in the hope that we could influence the subject to get long-term help.

A few subjects did not wish to come back for follow-up. We put a great deal of pressure on them to continue, using the trust we had previously established to motivate them. As clinicians we would have accepted their refusal; as researchers we almost never accepted a refusal without a great deal of persuasion. Our research assistant said after having called a subject three or four times to get them back, "I feel like I am a second rate salesman selling a third rate product." Here, too, the subjects' trust in us and their previous willingness to confide made this type of unsolicited persuasion more difficult for us. As doctors we would have preferred to leave them be.

The different abilities and means chosen by our probands to overcome childhood difficulties will be described via four selected longitudinal case histories.

▼ Case Vignettes: From Childhood to Adulthood

These case vignettes are selected to demonstrate diverse coping styles of individuals who continued to have symptoms of ADHD as adults, but who learned to function well, and who had found their own ways of overcoming their continued difficulties or using them constructively.

Jeffrey is a child we diagnosed and followed up with regular assessments between ages 5 and 25 years. At initial diagnosis his symptoms were aimless restlessness, difficulty focusing attention, and impulsivity. He was disliked by his peers because he was bossy and sometimes aggressive and would get into fights. He was also disobedient and had no fear of people in authority or of dangerous activities. By the time Jeffrey was in first grade he was slow to master reading, in spite of a WISC-R IQ of 133. Jeffrey at age 5 years (a year before he officially entered the longitudinal study) was treated with play therapy for 1 year, while his parents received counseling. The reason for this was that in addition to the above symptoms Jeffrey had a fascination for keys and would lift them out of others' pockets and collect them. Even in play therapy he managed to steal the therapist's keys out of her pocket, which she did not notice until she found she had no keys to get into her car. Jeffrey was sent to a sleep-away camp the summer he turned 6 years old (to give his parents a rest). They had given him (at his insistence) the keys to his trunk. Jeffrey was hysterical when he reached the camp and found he had lost his keys. He wanted to return home, but his mother drove 300 miles to bring replacements.

During adolescence, when undergoing one of his regular reassessments and while being tested by our research psychologist, Jeffrey revealed graphically that his fascination with keys was still a feature of his life. During his testing he pulled out handcuffs and before she could blink an eyelash, he had handcuffed the psychologist and locked the cuffs. She was ashamed to come out of the room handcuffed, and spent 30 minutes coaxing Jeffrey to unlock her. He finally did so. Jeffrey had a troubled adolescence and none of his symptoms abated. However, he never stole, did not abuse drugs or alcohol, was not violent or cruel. He had no friends, was behind in school, and was very disruptive in class to the point of getting himself expelled from two different public secondary schools. His parents, in desperation, found the funds for a private day school, and this turned out to be an important change. The principal of this school took a liking to Jeffrey, recognized his superior intelligence and spent a great deal of time after school hours with him, teaching him (among other things) how to read until he was at grade level. Although as an adult Jeffrey still never read for pleasure, he was able to complete a bachelor's degree in engineering and then a master's degree in burglar alarm systems. After graduation he moved out of Montreal and started his own burglar alarm company, which flourished. At the beginning of the company's existence Jeffrey would rush to the site of the burglary to tackle the burglar himself (he was allowed to carry a gun). One close shave in a gun fight finally ended Jeffrey's presence at the scene of the crime (his initial presence being a continued symptom of his childhood impulsivity and fearlessness).

Jeffrey taught us several things. His continued symptoms of ADHD were well channeled, as Jeffrey drove around all day long in his car with his cellular phone going constantly. His impulsivity and fearlessness at work were finally moderated when he faced real danger to his life, because he was almost shot. Earlier the presence of a "significant other" (the school principal) turned the tide of Jeffrey's long history of failure. Finally, his lifelong fascination with keys (whatever its origin) was channeled into a highly successful burglar alarm business.

Michael came to us for his first diagnosis of ADHD at age 6 years. He was a very likable, charming child, and at that age was accepted by peers. Unlike Jeffrey, his WISC-R IQ was average at 105, and he had significant specific learning disabilities and babyish speech. All through primary school he did poorly and was behind in reading, math, and spelling, and was in a special class for some subjects. In secondary school he was in a special school for children with learning disabilities. He dropped out of school in 10th grade at about an 8th grade standing. When Michael was 17 years old his parents moved to Hong Kong for business reasons. There Michael did odd jobs but none lasted longer than 2 or 3 months. His parents (both university graduates) became increasingly discouraged about the potential failure of their only son to find any way of supporting himself. A year later his father gave him a one-way ticket to Australia, and told Michael he could only come back when he had earned enough to pay back the fare.

In a large city suburb in Australia, Michael, aged 18 years, met Sally, who was 5 years older than he was and who had been orphaned. At age 23 years she had completed a degree in library science and had a stable job as a senior librarian. Their friendship solidified and soon they began living together. Sally encouraged Michael to get any kind of work, and Michael began to mow lawns, which he did well. With Sally's encouragement he stuck to this task until he was known and sought after; he soon purchased new equipment and hired others. This small business succeeded and Michael stayed at it for 3 years.

When he was 21 years old it was time for another assessment, and because we could not travel as far as Australia, we sent Michael all the forms for him to fill in. We did not hear anything for some time, and one day Michael and Sally turned up in my Montreal office.

"I wanted to tell you that your California Personality Inventory is crazy. No one in their right mind would answer 500 silly questions," said Michael.

"Is that why you came to see me?" I asked.

"Partly," he said, "just on a strong impulse I wanted to tell you that, so Sally and I decided to take a trip around the world to see you. I wanted you to meet Sally also."

Michael planned to stay awhile in Montreal and had managed to obtain a temporary work permit for Sally. This was very hard to do and when asked how he had succeeded, Michael replied, "I just told them I would marry Sally if they did not grant it, and if the marriage did not work out it would be their fault." (At that time if married to a Canadian Sally would be able to get a work permit without difficulty). Michael's old childhood charm had convinced the bureaucrats.

Michael's final assessment at age 26 years was a surprise. He had entered university as a mature student and obtained a degree in fine arts. Michael and Sally had been married for 4 years and ran a business. Sally organized Michael's work habits and was in charge of their social life. Friends liked Michael but although he alone did not keep his friends, as a couple they maintained close friends. Michael gave Sally his devoted admiration and loyalty and the two were getting along well. The mother role Sally had taken in the marriage changed when she was diagnosed to have breast cancer. The threat to Sally's health helped Michael to mature, and their relationship developed more mutual equality, although each gave different things to the other.

In our view, Michael and Sally were an example of Michael's marriage to a competent person resulting in his good adult outcome, in spite of the persistence of disability with respect to continuing symptoms of ADHD. The couple now have children and they continue to do well, although Sally has had to have renewed chemotherapy for recurrence of cancer.

John came in at age 6 years with symptoms of ADHD. He had no learning disability and no conduct or oppositional difficulties. Adolescence was a difficult time for him. It was a time when he began taking drugs, failing in school, and feeling hopeless about himself (to the point of being suicidal). A guidance counselor befriended him and prevented him from dropping out of secondary school. She intervened with the school system to save John from repeating a year, provided he took special remedial classes in the summer. In later adolescence, John's previous drug use led him to work in a drop-in center for adolescents who were taking drugs. He loved this work, and became so good at it that he was given a job in the psychiatric clinic of a teaching hospital to work with drug abusing adolescents. John did not finish high school but later managed to gain university entrance as a mature student. Because of continuing symptoms he flunked out of university, but finally, with the help of therapy and methylphenidate, he obtained his degree.

John's skill with helping others and his training for this as an adolescent gave him a head start. He is currently working at a senior level (as supervisor) in a large children's residential treatment center. John used his childhood adverse experiences and his understanding of children and adolescents to become superior in therapeutic skills. It was also interesting, in looking back over John's stages of development, that reading had always presented difficulties for him. At age 16 years he had become very concerned with civil rights issues of various kinds and had become an activist. At this time he wanted to read books to educate himself along political lines. With this heightened motivation he overcame reading difficulties; he is now an avid reader and plans eventually to complete his graduate studies. John is an example of an adult who used therapies well, including medication as an adult, and who turned his childhood difficulties into ways of understanding children and treating them. His case also provides another example of intervention on the part of a significant other—in John's case the guidance counselor who came into his life at a time of acute crisis and prevented him from dropping out of school, which in his then-suicidal mood might have led to a tragedy.

I hope that the preceding vignettes conveyed some of the richness, diversity, and drama that the subjects of our prospective, longitudinal study of hyperactive children illustrated. They did much to broaden our understanding and appreciation of how childhood pathology affects adult outcome, and how a great variety of factors, expected and unexpected, influence this outcome. We feel privileged that they shared their life stories with us. We hope the knowledge and understanding we have gained will help us develop more effective prevention and treatment approaches.

▼ Reference

Weiss G, Hechtman L: Hyperactive Children Grown Up. New York, Guilford, 1993

Index

*Page numbers printed in **boldface** type refer to tables or figures.*